Law in the Practice of Psychiatry

A HANDBOOK FOR CLINICIANS

CRITICAL ISSUES IN PSYCHIATRY
An Educational Series for Residents and Clinicians

Series Editor: **Sherwyn M. Woods, M.D., Ph.D.**
University of Southern California School of Medicine
Los Angeles, California

A RESIDENT'S GUIDE TO PSYCHIATRIC EDUCATION
Edited by Michael G. G. Thompson, M.D.

STATES OF MIND: Analysis of Change in Psychotherapy
Mardi J. Horowitz, M.D.

DRUG AND ALCOHOL ABUSE: A Clinical Guide to
Diagnosis and Treatment
Marc A. Schuckit, M.D.

**THE INTERFACE BETWEEN THE PSYCHODYNAMIC AND
BEHAVIORAL THERAPIES**
Edited by Judd Marmor, M.D. and Sherwyn M. Woods, M.D., Ph.D.

LAW IN THE PRACTICE OF PSYCHIATRY:
A Handbook for Clinicians
Seymour L. Halleck, M.D.

A Continuation Order Plan is available for this series. A continuation order will bring delivery of each new volume immediately upon publication. Volumes are billed only upon actual shipment. For further information please contact the publisher.

Law in the Practice of Psychiatry

A HANDBOOK FOR CLINICIANS

Seymour L. Halleck, M.D.

University of North Carolina
Chapel Hill, North Carolina

With the Assistance of

Nancy H. Halleck, J.D.

Plenum Medical Book Company · New York and London

ISBN 0-306-40373-0

©1980 Plenum Publishing Corporation
227 West 17th Street, New York, N.Y. 10011

Plenum Medical Book Company is an imprint of Plenum Publishing Corporation

Printed in the United States of America

To Dr. Karl A. Menninger
who taught so many so much about
psychiatry, law, and life

Foreword

Once upon a time only forensic psychiatrists had much to do with law and the legal system. Now, hardly a day passes in the life of a clinician without some significant encounter with the interface between the law and the practice of psychiatry. That interface extends all the way from the general regulation of clinical practice to the specifics of clinical management of individual patients. It includes, like the chapters of this book, such important topics as informed consent, right to treatment, privilege and confidentiality, patients' rights, competency, psychiatric testimony, malpractice, and liability.

Dr. Halleck is one of the professions' most distinguished thinkers and authors in the field of psychiatry and law, and is this year's recipient of the coveted Isaac Ray Award of the American Psychiatric Association. Having spent his entire academic and professional life deeply involved in the clinical practice of psychiatry, he is particularly well suited to understand and respond to the clinician's need for a clear and concise elucidation of those areas of psychiatry and law which are involved in the daily work of psychiatrists and all mental health professionals.

Dr. Halleck approaches his task in a novel question and answer format. The result is a book that is not only relevant and practical, but eminently readable. It not only defines the limits of ethical and legal practice, but enables us to make better use of the legal system for the benefit of our patients, and to avoid the anguish of unnecessary litigation and malpractice lawsuits. This is the sort of book that one keeps close at hand for regular consultation. It is a most welcome addition to this series, "Critical Issues in Psychiatry."

Sherwyn M. Woods, M.D., Ph.D.

Preface

This book is written for clinicians and for those training to be clinicians. The legal questions it raises and seeks to answer are those which have become of increasing concern to me, my colleagues, and my students in day-to-day practice. Some of the issues could undoubtedly have been formulated with greater erudition if I had asked attorneys to contribute directly to the writing, but I felt from the beginning of this project that I would serve my audience best by maintaining the perspective of a clinician throughout and by keeping legal issues as uncomplicated and as psychiatrically relevant as I possibly could.

Even though legal issues are not elaborated here in great depth, I could not possibly have presented them adequately without the assistance of attorneys. My daughter, Nancy Halleck, was my primary legal collaborator. She helped me collect cases, guided me through the malpractice literature, and corrected errors of law I made in initial drafts. Two professors with whom I have had the privilege of conjointly teaching mental health law were also extremely helpful. Alexander Brooks, Professor of Law at Rutgers University and the winner of the Guttmacher Award in 1975, provided me with excellent advice and encouragement. Barry Nakell, Professor of Law at the University of North Carolina, has through the years helped clarify many legal issues for me, has kept me informed of new opinions, and has always been available to answer my questions.

I am also endebted to Sherwyn Woods and Hilary Evans who repeatedly encouraged me when I felt overwhelmed by the task of writing a text which goes beyond my own specialty training. And finally, Mary Lou Allison and Danna Menzaco made my task so much easier by typing the many drafts of the text and by helping with its organization.

This is also an appropriate place to offer a word of caution and a brief apology. While most legal issues relevant to psychiatry are discussed here, the reader who is involved in actual litigation cannot use this book as a substitute for obtaining legal counsel. For a variety of reasons, which will be expanded upon in the text, the psychiatrist is well advised to consult with an attorney whenever there is legal risk to the patient or risk of malpractice. My apology is for the use of discriminatory language. In the interest of brevity I have used the traditional "he" and "him" rather than more cumbersome neutral terms.

Seymour L. Halleck

Contents

Introduction
Psychiatry and Law
—General Issues

The practice of psychiatry is in large part regulated by law, but this is a relatively recent development. Up until the mid-1960s the law made few demands on us. Our day-to-day practice was not heavily monitored by government agencies, nor did negative outcomes in treating patients put us in jeopardy of being sued for malpractice. Before legal regulation of psychiatry expanded so rapidly, psychiatrists viewed their relationship to the law as one in which they provided valuable assistance. The law allowed psychiatrists to assist society in the social control function of restraining and treating deviant and disorderly people. We were given considerable power to define our own role in managing the behavior of the mentally ill, and for the most part society appreciated our efforts. The courts also asked psychiatrists for assistance in resolving conflicts which were influenced by the mental status of one or both parties in litigation. Here the psychiatrist was expected to be an expert witness. Few psychiatrists volunteered to be expert witnesses, but when they did their services were usually welcomed.

Today the legal system makes different demands of the psychiatrist, which are not easily met. The new changes influence the manner in which we provide direct care of patients. Over the past decade we have lost much of our freedom to choose how we will treat patients. Like other doctors, our activities are increasingly regulated by state and federal agencies. By regulating third-party payment, federal agencies (as well as private insurers) manipulate the rewards or reinforcement provided to doctors so as to shape their practices in conformity with acceptable standards. The legal system has also significantly expanded the frequency and extent of punishment for practicing in a negligent manner. Malpractice lawsuits are increasing in all branches of medicine. But psychiatry, which was once thought of as a specialty almost immune from lawsuits, has become a more common target for malpractice litigation. There has been an even more profound change in the psychiatrist's role in dealing with the severely mentally ill. Psychiatrists have lost much of their power to act independently in controlling the behavior of severely disturbed patients. Our courts have accepted the proposition that unmonitored psychiatric treatment of people who behave in a disturbed manner may lead to violations of their civil rights. This has spawned a great deal of litigation and legislation which massively curtails the psychiatrist's capacity to function autonomously in dealing with nonconsenting patients.

The least dramatic changes have occurred with regard to the role of the psychiatrist as expert witness. There has been some expansion of the use of psychiatric testimony to help resolve a wide variety of legal and social issues, but this expansion has not had a major impact on the daily practice of psychiatry. It is still true that only a relatively small proportion of psychiatrists testify in court as experts on such issues as competency to stand trial, criminal insanity, competency to make a will, or the determination of child custody.

Because of society's new regulation of the activities of psychiatrists, it is becoming difficult for a psychiatrist to practice from day to day without some knowledge of what the law expects of him. The days of laissez-faire practice are gone. It is still possible to practice effective and humane psychiatry, but it is no longer possible to treat certain types of patients effectively without consideration of legal issues. Often treatment cannot even be instituted without the approval of judicial agencies. The rules by which psychiatry deals with nonconsenting patients have been changed so drastically that failure to have considerable awareness of current law may put the psychiatrist in jeopardy of a civil suit. In my own practice, which consists largely of treating both voluntary and involuntary inpatients in a university hospital setting, I find that I must spend as much as 20% of my clinical time dealing with and teaching about issues which involve the law. Some psychiatrists have structured their practices in a way which allows them to be less preoccupied with legal issues, but no psychiatrist is unaffected by legal issues in daily practice.

This book is designed to assist the practicing psychiatrist and psychiatric resident in dealing with issues related to psychiatry and law. The first two parts are a simplified description of how psychiatric practice is currently regulated by law. The third part is a discussion of the role of the psychiatrist as an expert witness. The role of the expert may not be a day-to-day concern of the average practicing psychiatrist, but it is likely that more than once in his professional lifetime the psychiatrist will assume the role of expert in relationship to the courts. Even the psychiatrist who never intends to assume the expert role should know something about it. Most of the social conflicts we are asked to help resolve have some relevance to psychiatry. They raise fascinating questions, the study of which can expand our understanding of human behavior. We should also be aware that the public image of psychiatry is largely determined by the manner in which we or our colleagues perform as courtroom experts.

Until recently, most of the writing about psychiatry and law has focused on expert witness roles. One common theme in much of this writing is the need for the two professions to cooperate with one another. Psychiatrists often have views quite different from lawyers as to how certain social conflicts are best conceptualized and resolved. If both professions are to participate in processes of conflict resolution, it makes sense for them to understand one another's viewpoints and to seek a common base of understanding. It is relatively easy for the psychiatrist to adopt a cooperative stance while in the expert role. Experts do not have any direct stake in the decision of a court and only their ideologies and egos are threatened by what they consider an adverse ruling. Our willingness to cooperate with the legal profession is inherent in the voluntary nature of our participation in the expert role. We are in the courts to help the legal system and we can remove ourselves from the process whenever we wish.

It should be clear, however, that when we are not experts but are subject to the new legal regulation of psychiatric practice, the issues of conflict and cooperation with the law take on a different meaning. Here we are not above the conflict: we are part of the conflict. We are not voluntary actors in the legal process, but involuntary clients whose participation can be psychologically and financially costly. Not only are our ideologies and egos at stake, but we can also lose our freedom to choose how we will practice medicine and control our wealth. Like involuntary participants in any process, our cooperation is grudging. Because of the voluntary nature of psychiatrists' involvement as experts in the early development of forensic psychiatry, some psychiatrists still have a picture of psychiatry's relationship to the law as one in which forces of equal power either battle or work together. In considering the current legal regulation of psychiatry, this is a false image. (For that matter, it was probably a false image even twenty years ago. In my opinion, psychiatrists have always overestimated their impact on the legal system.) It may also be a highly maladaptive image insofar as it prevents us from behaving realistically.

Our capacity to influence the outcome of litigation in which we have a professional interest or are one of the adversaries is limited. Psychiatrists have no more power in courtroom proceedings than any other witnesses or defendants. Outside of the courtroom we have the same prerogatives as any other concerned group: we can object to legal rulings, we can try to educate the public and the legal profession as to deficiencies of legal rulings, and we can even initiate litigation which might change legal rulings. But we must divest ourselves of grandiosity. In confronting the reality of legal regulation of our practices, our cooperation is often involuntary and we must deal with the regulators from a defensive posture.

The Changing Nature of Law

No matter how vehemently psychiatrists may oppose current legal changes, they will want to obey the law. An immediate problem here is that it is not always clear what the law expects from us. The two chief sources of law are statutes and precedents. Statutes are laws made by legislatures which consist of elected representatives of the people. Statutes differ from state to state and, as will be noted repeatedly, statutes which govern various aspects of psychiatric practice are no exception. The statutes enacted by the various states must also be legal under the Constitution of the United States. Thus, even a law enacted by a state legislature may be found unconstitutional and illegal by higher federal courts, by state Supreme Courts, or by the Supreme Court of the United States.

Precedents come from courts, and to a lesser extent from administrative bodies of government. Law is created by precedent when courts make decisions or take actions that serve as a rule for future determinations in similar or related cases. When a court decides on a given case, certain rules and principles are enunciated to justify that decision. These rules and principles are then applicable to new cases. Once a question of law has been deliberately examined and decided in a United States court, it is binding on that court's jurisdiction. Other jurisdictions will also take note of that decision and may use it to help resolve similar conflicts. The development of law through precedents provides stability to the legal system. When faced with a legal conflict there is usually some similar situation which has been adjudicated to turn to. Law developed through precedents can also be flexible: as social conditions and social attitudes change, old precedents are regularly modified and new ones are developed.

Much of the law in the United States is derived from judicial decisions based on usage and customs of antiquity which became principles recognized in the ancient unwritten law of England. This law is not codified, but is a collection of precedents reflecting the judicial wisdom of centuries of litigation. Collectively, these precedents are referred to as common law. The common law is the basic source of law in all states except Louisiana.

Precedents are created and utilized by both state and federal courts. In the state system, legal actions or proceedings usually begin in lower courts or courts of original jurisdiction. Courts of general or superior jurisdiction hear more serious cases and also serve as courts of appeal. A superior court can overrule the findings of a court of original jurisdiction. The process of appealing a decision to a higher court is, however, quite complicated and governed by strict procedures. The federal judicial system includes district courts, circuit courts of appeal, and the Supreme Court of the United States. There is also a hierarchy here in which a superior court can overrule the findings of a lesser court. As in state courts, strict criteria are used to determine which cases can be appealed. In both state and federal systems, the decision of the higher court is binding on all lesser courts within its jurisdiction.

There are limits to the type of cases that can be brought before a federal court and there are rules governing the bringing of an appeal from a state court to a federal court. Federal district courts hear cases which involve disputes between citizens of different states, between citizens and aliens, and questions which arise under the Constitution of the United States. (There are other areas of litigation such as those involving copyrights and internal revenues which are handled directly by federal courts.) Generally, federal courts will consider appeals from state courts only when federal or constitutional questions are involved. It should be apparent from the above material that the legal system in the United States is a complex set of structures and that the law varies with locality.

The law also varies rapidly over time and is constantly being revised. Currently, there are many decisions which affect psychiatry that have been adjudicated in state or lower federal courts and are now being appealed to higher courts. The law in these instances will change if the higher courts overrule the lower courts. In this era of massive litigation the law may even vary on a day-to-day basis.

Thus, the law rarely provides definitive answers to general questions. The psychiatrist who asks questions such as "Can I initiate commitment of nondangerous patients?" "Do patients have a right to be treated?" and "Do patients have a right to refuse treatment?" can expect inconclusive answers or answers which are likely to be relevant to only a particular locality at a particular point in time. This complicates enormously the task of the psychiatrist who wishes to keep abreast of legal issues. There is never any ultimate source that can provide an up-to-date picture of the law. Even efforts to keep abreast of current developments by reading journals and periodicals may result in confusion, since court decisions which receive a lot of publicity are often relevant only to a particular area of the country or to one particular type of case.

The prediction of the law's response to specific questions is also a matter of great uncertainty. Sometimes precedents relevant to a given case may conflict with one another. Changing social conditions also motivate the courts to view some precedents as irrelevant and to create new precedents. A court's response to a particular case will also vary with the facts of the case. The same court may rule that a patient who presents a certain picture of mental illness and dangerousness is commitable but that another patient whose clinical picture is only slightly different is not. Predicting the response of the legal system is particularly difficult when the statutory law in the related area is vague. Many of the statutes which govern psychiatric treatment are phrased in terms which are poorly defined and ambiguous. These statutes are subject to a variety of interpretations. Finally, our constitution is itself subject to a variety of interpretations and the higher federal courts and the Supreme Court may base their rulings on interpretations which are influenced by changing social conditions.

In the area of malpractice, it is especially difficult for a psychiatrist to have a clear idea as to which types of errors, or bad results, will lead to successful malpractice suits and which will not. Gross negligence or gross abuse of the patient, of course, is always actionable, but many suits are brought and won in situations where the wrongfulness of the physician's behavior is not readily apparent. Malpractice law is governed primarily by the common law, and the rules of law in malpractice suits do not have a consistent influence in determining the final decision. In this area much unfettered discretion is left to the judge and jury. The psychological response of the judge or jury members to the facts of a given case may, for example, play a critical role in their decision. Even when the rules of malpractice in a given case would seem to indicate that a physician is blameless, it is not unheard of for a jury to award damages to a plaintiff who is viewed as having a sympathetic case. The physician faced with a question regarding malpractice cannot expect a clear answer from an attorney as to how that issue would be resolved if litigated. Usually the attorney can provide only an educated guess.

Over my years of practice I have often heard colleagues ask "What is the law on this subject?" Many psychiatrists assume that this question is readily answerable and that the answer will tell how a given legal problem is likely to be resolved. Such an assumption as to the exactness or predictability of the law is naive. The practice of law, like much of the practice of medicine and life itself, is plagued by uncertainty. Predictions as to outcomes of legal disputes are at best probability statements.

Psychiatrists will live more comfortably and deal more effectively with changing legal standards if they have a greater appreciation of the purposes of law and the kind of thinking that dominates resolution of legal conflict. The object of law is to enforce standards of social behavior and to provide rules which allow for a kind of fair interaction between individuals and groups and which lessen the probability of conflict. Where conflict cannot be avoided, the law provides a means of adjudication or peaceful settlement through the instrumentality of the courts. In setting standards and resolving conflicts, the law attempts to define patterns of behavior which are deemed right by the society. Through law, each culture defines its ideal image of morality and justice.

A lawsuit brought before a court is a proceeding designed to settle a controversy between two or more persons. It is always adversarial. Each participant in the courtroom struggle has a goal which cannot be satisfied without imposing a sense of loss upon the other. The legal proceeding is similar to a "zero sum" game in which one side loses and one side wins. It is not a scientific procedure in which the search for truth leads to the examination of all relevant data and to the testing of all reasonable hypotheses. Legal proceedings do not afford the opportunity for a leisurely pursuit of knowledge. Considerations of morality and justice require the court to make a decision which will impute or deny blame as quickly as possible. Even though its decisions may have powerful and far-reaching consequences, there is little opportunity for the court to equivocate. A defendant is guilty or not guilty. A defendant is liable or not liable.

Psychiatrists naturally have difficulty in appreciating the kind of thinking that goes into legal decision-making. As scientists, we are committed primarily to the search for truth. We are trained to consider all possible hypotheses and to search out all relevant facts. As scientists, we assume responsibility for considering the weaknesses of our hypotheses as well as their strengths. The possibility of arriving at truth through procedures in which each party to a conflict presents only arguments which favor its case and deliberately deletes arguments which weaken its case is alien to us. Psychiatrists are also uncomfortable in viewing one answer as the definitive resolution of a problem. Ordinarily, we view any given act as being determined by a wide variety of factors. We are rarely forced to make conclusive decisions when our data are inconclusive. More commonly, we have the luxury of experimenting with interventions that do not produce irrevocable consequences.

It is my experience that few doctors appreciate why the legal system has adopted the type of reasoning and procedures it uses in its effort to dispense justice. Nevertheless, psychiatrists must learn to accept the reality that decision-making in the courtroom is not likely to be governed by the same intellectual methods that are involved in discovering new medical facts or treating patients. When we enter the courtroom, we become involved in someone else's "ball-game" and must play by his rules. It is futile to recriminate against the unscientific nature of these rules. A certain amount of trust in a system that has served our country well for over two centuries seems warranted.

Although I believe that psychiatrists will fare better in dealing with the law if they adopt a dispassionate approach to the legal system, I am well aware of the enormous impact that recent legal changes have had on our profession. Psychiatry views itself as a profession under legal attack, and with good reason. Actions we once took automatically as proper and necessary aspects of treatment may now be viewed as illegal assaults upon the patient. Psychiatrists are frequently depicted in the legal literature as people who have too much power and who abuse that power by arbitrarily depriving patients of their constitutional rights. Sometimes we face charges that our work is dangerous or ineffective or both. There are a considerable number of attorneys who sincerely believe these charges. It is not easy for psychiatrists who view themselves as people who wish to remedy human suffering to find themselves viewed as people who cause human suffering.

The greatest frustration created by the new legalism, however, is the manner in which it prevents us from doing what we believe is best for patients. These days the psychiatrist often encounters patients who will benefit from a certain type of treatment, but finds that new laws make the use of such treatment difficult or impossible to implement. Complex legal procedures sometimes replace the authority of the doctor in determining whether certain forms of treatment can be used. Often these procedures are so complicated and time-consuming that only the doctor who works with a well-staffed organization can afford to take the time to see that treatment is implemented. There is nothing quite so demoralizing to a doctor as watching a patient who is obviously treatable refuse treatment, leave the hospital, and continue to inflict more suffering upon himself and his loved ones.

The rise in the number of medical malpractice suits has also, in my opinion, had some adverse effects on the quality of psychiatric practice. Psychiatrists, like all other doctors, now spend a considerable amount of time filling out forms and putting extensive notes in charts largely to shield themselves from litigation. This consumes time that might have been spent with patients. Like other doctors, we also respond to the threat of malpractice by practicing defensively. We order too many tests and keep patients hospitalized too long (or, conversely, sometimes discharge patients too soon) in order to be safe from the threat of a malpractice suit. One of the first things the young resident learns on a psychiatric inpatient unit is to "cover himself," namely, to make sure that nothing is done to the patient that will make the doctor or the hospital liable for malpractice. Such a preoccupation has become an integral part of psychiatric training and practice.

Psychiatrists are certainly not unanimous in their disillusionment with recent legal changes. Some psychiatrists welcome a few of the changes and a few psychiatrists may welcome all of them. We are aware that when our practices were unmonitored, a small but significant number of patients were badly damaged by being deprived of their rights. We are also aware that the increase in malpractice litigation may be forcing us to take a much-needed look at our standards of diagnosis and treatment. Many of us who are highly committed to civil liberties have at times even welcomed the intrusions of the courts. My residents, who often begin psychiatric training with a civil-libertarian orientation and a profound distaste for participating in any involuntary commitment proceedings, often ask me if I believe the new legalism has been good or bad for patients. My response is that it has certainly been good for patients treated in institutions with inadequate facilities and for patients treated by incompetent doctors. But at the same time, it has probably diminished the quality of care that adequate facilities and competent doctors can provide their patients. Over all, I fear that more patients have been hurt by the new legalism than have been helped by it.

My residents usually do not ask whether the degree of satisfaction psychiatrists derive from their practice has been more or less since the advent of the new legalism because the answer here is obvious. Unless the psychiatrist has a deep intellectual interest in forensic issues, the legal regulation of our activities makes practice far less rewarding than it used to be.

One way of conceptualizing our professional dilemma is in terms of the differing expectations being put on us on the one hand by statutory law and the rulings of federal courts and on the other hand by malpractice law. New statutes and new declaratory judgments and injunctions coming from the federal courts have curtailed significantly the power of the psychiatrist in dealing with patients. At the same time, new rulings in tort or malpractice law seem to be expanding the psychiatrist's responsibility for patients. We have less power to treat patients the way we want to, but we are increasingly held responsible for bad outcomes of treatment, and even for some of the consequences of our patients' actions. Any group of people who are being given increasing responsibility for outcomes which they have less power to control will perceive themselves as oppressed. In relationship to the legal system, psychiatrists now perceive themselves as an oppressed group.

Ultimately, one of the most depressing consequences of the new legalism is that it discourages psychiatrists from working with the sickest patients. Throughout much of this century, one of the most troubling aspects of psychiatric practice in this country has been that psychiatrists receive the greatest financial and status rewards when they work with healthier patients and avoid more disturbed patients. Unfortunately, the best resources of the psychiatric profession have been concentrated on those who are least ill. The new legalism accelerates this trend. Much of the litigation involving psychiatry in the last fifteen years has centered around the highly disturbed, the violent, and the institutionalized patient. By avoiding such patients, the psychiatrist can spare himself the formidable stress of wasted hours doing the legal paperwork required by new rulings and worrying about malpractice suits. There is now less incentive than ever for a psychiatrist to work with severely disturbed patients. If our society does not soon come up with a new reward system for encouraging a renewed commitment to such patients, their plight will continue to worsen.

For the moment, psychiatrists have no alternative but to accommodate to the changes brought about by the new legalism. One purpose of the first two sections of this book is to delineate ways in which such accommodation can take place. At the same time as we are obeying the law, however, we have a right to inform members of the legal system and other citizens as to errors we perceive in current legalistic approaches. To the extent that our critiques and dissent are knowledgeable, they are more likely to have an impact on those who monitor our practices. A second purpose in the first two parts of the book, then, is to expand the reader's knowledge of conceptual issues involved in control of psychiatric practice. Such an analysis should help delineate the rights as well as the obligations of the practicing psychiatrist. It should strengthen the psychiatrist's position as an advocate of rational mental health law.

PART I
MALPRACTICE

1

Medical Malpractice Law and the Psychiatrist

The threat of being sued for malpractice exerts a relatively consistent and powerful influence on every physician. No matter how it is resolved, a malpractice suit is a substantial source of punishment for the doctor. It is always time-consuming. If the doctor feels he has done no wrong, there is no way he can avoid powerful feelings of anger toward the plaintiff and the plaintiff's attorney. If he feels that he may have done wrong, he must deal with painful feelings of self-recrimination. Malpractice suits may drag on for years. During this time the physician will be haunted by the possibility of an adverse judgment that might result in loss of professional prestige, higher liability insurance premiums, cancellation of insurance, legal fees not covered by insurance, or even a financially devastating judgment in excess of insurance coverage.

Malpractice law is primarily designed to provide a just means of compensating victims of poor medical practice.[1] But it also serves an educational or deterrent function for physicians.[2] The physician who is sued for negligent practice will supposedly improve his future standards of practice. Other physicians will be deterred from negligent practice by observing the plight of the physician defendant. In this sense, malpractice law as it relates to the physician can be viewed as supplementing or extending the criminal law. It regulates the physician's behavior by posing a constant threat of punishment for unacceptable behavior.

Malpractice law also helps to define standards of practice. Ideally, decisions coming from the courts should help clarify what is acceptable and what is unacceptable practice. In a sense the courts serve to confirm

---

[1]W. Prosser, *The Law of Torts,* 4th ed. (St. Paul; Minn.: West, 1971).
[2]A. R. Morris and C. R. Morris, *Handbook of Legal Medicine* (St. Louis: C. V. Mosby, 1970).

or validate professional standards. The equity of this process, however, is questionable.

Legal writers assert repeatedly that if the physician practices in a manner that would be affirmed as acceptable by the standards of his profession, he will not be liable for malpractice.[3] Practicing physicians, however, believe that there are exceptions to such statements. Many physicians fear that they can be punished by malpractice suits in an arbitrary and capricious manner.[4] In psychiatry there are times when doing what most colleagues would judge to be best for the patient may leave the psychiatrist in a vulnerable legal position. Sometimes the psychiatrist must make judgments as to how much risk of malpractice he is willing to incur in order to act in a manner he believes is best for his patient.

Under What Legal Doctrines Are Suits Brought against Psychiatrists?

Most civil actions against physicians are brought under the law of torts. A part of the common law and based on precedents, tort law is uncodified and in large part unaffected by statute. A tort is a civil wrong other than a breach of contract for which one may have a remedy in the form of an action for damages. Another way of defining a tort is as an action by a person harmful to another person that the law recognizes and for which it provides a legal method to stop that harm or correct the damage. In order to be charged with legal responsibility for a tort, one must be at fault; that is, one must have committed an intentional wrong or have been negligent. If the physician harms a patient, either intentionally or by negligence, he may be sued.[5]

Although the physician–patient relationship is essentially based on an implied contract, the physician usually does not guarantee or promise definitive results. Traditionally, the law of contracts has played an insignificant role in medical malpractice.[6] Poor results may occur in medical practice even with the best possible care. There is, therefore, a time-honored axiom in the common law that the liability of a physician cannot be based solely on the fact of unsuccessful treatment. The successful suits of physicians for breach of contract have occurred in situations where

[3]D. M. Harney, *Medical Malpractice* (Indianapolis: Allen Smith, 1973); J. R. Waltz and F. E. Inbau, *Medical Jurisprudence* (New York: Macmillan, 1971).
[4]L. Berlin, "Malpractice: Doctors Have a Right to Make Mistakes," *Medical Economics*, Feb. 6, 1978, pp. 165–72.
[5]A. R. Holder, *Medical Malpractice Law* (New York: Wiley, 1975); A. R. Rosenberg and L. S. Goldsmith, *Malpractice Made Easy* (New York: Books for Industry, 1976).
[6]H. J. King, *The Law of Medical Malpractice in a Nutshell* (St. Paul, Minn.: West, 1977).

the physician promised or guaranteed results.[7] Gynecologists, urologists, or general surgeons who perform sterilization operations, for example, have successfully been sued when they guaranteed results and the patient or the patient's spouse later became pregnant. Suits involving breach of contract can be financially disastrous for the physician since many malpractice policies do not cover this cause of legal action.

There are no recorded cases of a psychiatrist's being sued for breach of contract. This does not mean, however, that such suits will never occur or have not occurred and were settled out of court. Therapists who demand payment in advance are likely to promise certain results and thereby put themselves in a vulnerable position. A more common area of potential concern involves the clinician's use of reassurance. While only the most rash psychiatrist routinely promises favorable results at the beginning of treatment, many psychiatrists are prone to be excessively reassuring in dealing with certain kinds of patients. It is often useful, for example, to remind depressed patients that depression is a reversible disorder and that there is every likelihood that they will get well. I have on more than one occasion guaranteed a severely depressed and agitated patient that he would recover. Clinically, this is a useful technique which in some instances buoys the hopes of the distraught patient and spares him needless suffering. As I have learned more about malpractice law, however, I have come to appreciate the legal riskiness of this technique. If these patients had not recovered, I might have been liable for breach of contract. Prudent psychiatrists might want to couch their reassurances in probability terms. It is safer to tell the patient "the great majority of patients recover from this condition" than to say "there is no doubt you will get better." This is one instance in which a kind of emphatic reassurance which involves a promise might be the best possible treatment for the patient, yet it might put the psychiatrist in jeopardy of a lawsuit.

Dr. Ralph Slovenko, one of the most eminent scholars in the field of legal psychiatry, has argued recently that we may eventually see malpractice suits being litigated under contract rather than tort law.[8] He notes that it is extremely difficult to define negligent conduct in psychiatry and that some remedy must be available to those who do not respond to psychotherapy. He argues further that medicine has become indistinguishable from a commercial enterprise and therefore should be subject to the same kind of legal actions that govern commerce. Slovenko's view is interesting, but highly controversial. The majority of

---

[7]*Guilmet v. Campbell,* 385 Mich. 57, 188 N.W. 2d 601 (1971).
[8]R. Slovenko, " 'Mal-Psychotherapy' Suits May Soon Beset Psychiatrists," *Roche Reports, Frontiers of Psychiatry, 8* (March 1, 1978): 5.

scholars in this area see no immediate shift from tort to contract law in the regulation of malpractice.

There is one more legal doctrine under which a psychiatrist could, in theory, be sued. Under the doctrine of strict liability, an individual who engages in an activity that harms others may be morally blameless but nevertheless legally at fault. Certain activities such as storing dangerous substances are socially useful or necessary, but inherently dangerous. If harm results from such activities, a suit is possible. It has been argued that psychotherapy is an inherently dangerous activity and that psychiatrists should be sued for bad results even if their intentions are noble and they are not negligent.[9] Such a theory is not, of course, taken seriously by the majority of legal scholars.

What Is the Likelihood of a Psychiatrist's Being Sued for Malpractice?

It is not easy to find out how frequently psychiatrists are sued for malpractice. Many cases are settled out of court and some are settled in courts which do not publish records. It is possible to get some idea of the nature of suits by studying only recorded cases, but this does not give an adequate index of frequency. Furthermore, decisions made in courts of record may not accurately reflect the nature of litigation which is influencing the average practitioner. A more informative means of determining how malpractice claims are affecting the average practitioner is to survey the medical malpractice claims files of insurance companies. Such surveys are published infrequently and do not reflect claims for uninsured physicians or for tortious actions which are not insured. A third and probably the most informative means of assessing frequency simply involves surveying psychiatrists and asking them about their own involvement in malpractice suits during a given period of time. The value of this method is, of course, dependent on the extent of cooperation of the parties surveyed.

Whichever method of data collection is employed, there is general agreement that psychiatrists are sued far less frequently than most other physicians, but that the number of suits against psychiatrists is rising at a rate which is faster than that of other specialties.[10] One of the better-known studies concluded that a psychiatrist can expect to be sued once every fifty to one hundred years as compared to the average for all

[9]C. Kennedy, "Comment: Injuries Precipitated by Psychotherapy: Liability Without Fault as a Basis for Recovery," *South Dakota Law Review*, 20, no. 2 (1975): 401–17.

[10]H. L. Hirsch and E. R. White, "Why Do Patients Sue? The Pathologic Anatomy of Medical Malpractice Claims," *Legal Aspects of Medical Practice* 6, no. 1 (1978): 25–32.

doctors of once every seven years.[11] Another more recent study concluded that a suit against a psychiatrist is likely to occur every twenty-five to seventy-five years.[12]

The nature of the psychiatrist's practice has some relationship to his susceptibility to a lawsuit. Psychiatrists who hospitalize patients, who prescribe medication frequently, and who use electroconvulsive therapy are at greater risk of being sued than those who do not.[13] There are also geographical variables involved in the incidence of malpractice suits. Urbanized states have a higher rate of malpractice claims than rural states. This is important to the psychiatric profession since so many psychiatrists practice in urban areas. It is also of interest that the western part of the country has the largest number of suits. The East has slightly fewer and the South has the least.

There is general agreement among observers in the malpractice field that the increase in litigation against doctors is related to the following factors:

1. There are many new procedures in medicine which require greater skills and knowledge. Possibilities of negligence expand as more is expected of the physician.
2. Patients seem to have developed greater expectations of their physicians. The public is very claims conscious, and more people have developed a sophisticated view of medical activities from popular literature and other media.
3. As medical practice becomes more technical, there has been considerable diminution of rapport between patient and doctor. A large number of malpractice claims are initiated after the physician turns his bill over to a collection agency and the patient responds indignantly with a lawsuit.[14]
4. There are many more lawyers in this country now and the competitive nature of legal practice encourages them to develop new areas of litigation. There is a tendency for malpractice cases to increase in states which have developed no-fault auto insurance practices. Conceivably, when attorneys are limited in opportunity to gain awards in one area, they may simply focus on another. The contingency fee system in which the attorney re-

[11]C. L. Trent and W. P. Muhl, "Professional Liability Insurance and the American Psychiatrist," *American Journal of Psychiatry* 132 (1975): 1312-14.
[12]P. F. Slawson, "Psychiatric Malpractice: A California State Wide Survey," *Bulletin of the American Academy of Psychiatry and the Law 6*, (1978): 58-63.
[13]P. F. Slawson, "Psychiatric Malpractice: The California Experience," *Proceedings of the American Psychiatric Association,* 1978, p. 141 (summary).
[14]W. A. Bellamy, "Psychiatric Malpractice," in *American Handbook of Psychiatry,* edited by S. Arieti (New York: Basic Books, 1975), vol. 5, chap. 45.

ceives a percentage of the award if the patient wins and nothing if the patient loses may encourage both plaintiffs and attorneys to initiate and press more suits. Plaintiffs have little to lose in initiating suits and attorneys have much to gain in vigorously pressing suits.

5. As medical practice becomes more complicated, doctors employ more assistants and may be liable for the negligent actions of their employees. Attending physicians in educational settings are particularly vulnerable if they are not sufficiently diligent in supervising the work of interns and residents.

There are certain aspects of psychiatric practice which may discourage malpractice litigation. As will be noted in more detail later, there is no ground for malpractice unless acceptable standards of diagnosis and treatment are breached. Such standards are obviously difficult to define in psychiatry. Psychiatric patients may also be less eager to institute suits since litigation may require them to reveal intimate details of their personal lives. Furthermore, most patients have positive feelings toward their psychiatrists and remain loyal even when the outcome of treatment is clearly unfavorable. Psychiatrists, more than other medical practitioners, take the time to listen to their patients and are skilled in dealing with the patient's hostile and negative feelings.

As psychiatrists move closer to practicing under a more traditional medical model, they are likely to be subjected to more frequent malpractice claims. Some authorities believe that much of the recent litigation against psychiatrists is related to our more frequent use of drugs and other biological treatments.[15] It is possible that in our recent reaffirmation of the medical model, we are adopting some of its worst aspects and are failing to pay sufficient attention to our personal relationship with patients. The move to a more biological psychiatry may not, however, be a sufficient explanation of the increase in psychiatric malpractice cases. Another possible explanation is that some of the new civil rights legislation puts restrictions on psychiatrists of which they may be unaware. Psychiatrists may be sued for violating a patient's civil rights even when they believe they are following, and are protected by, state law.[16] It is also possible that some of the less conventional and more controversial experiential psychotherapies which are currently popular may put practitioners at greater risk of a lawsuit. These therapies involve a great deal

[15]S. E. Fishalow, "The Tort Liability of the Psychiatrist," *Bulletin of the American Academy of Psychiatry and the Law 3*, no. 4 (1975): 191–224.

[16]A. S. Stone, "The Commission on Judicial Action of the American Psychiatric Association: Origins and Prospects—A Personal View," *Bulletin of the American Academy of Psychiatry and Law 3*, no. 3 (1975): 119.

of traumatic self-disclosure and physical contact. They can increase the risk of actual or perceived harm to the patient.

What Should a Psychiatrist Do When Informed That He Is Being Sued for Malpractice?

The actions to be taken in response to the notice in the form of a summons and complaint that a suit has been filed are routine and straightforward. In most instances the psychiatrist will carry malpractice insurance and the first action to take is to inform the insurance carrier of the petition. The carrier will probably require the filing of a report of the incident on which the malpractice is allegedly based. The psychiatrist is then likely to be interviewed by representatives of the insurance company and its attorneys. If the psychiatrist is not covered by malpractice insurance, if the amount of damages requested in the complaint exceeds the amount of insurance coverage, or if the particular allegation involves a tort which is not covered in the psychiatrist's policy, the psychiatrist should immediately hire his own attorney. The procedures of the litigation process (which will be elaborated in more detail later) are incredibly complicated. None but the most legally sophisticated physician could hope to defend himself without an attorney, and there should never be hesitation in obtaining legal help, either independently or through the insurance carrier. Obviously, complete candor and cooperation with one's attorney are essential.

It is well to ascertain at this point that all records pertaining to the patient and the particular incident related to the suit are available and in a safe place. These records should be reviewed very carefully so that the psychiatrist can provide the most effective cooperation with the attorney. It should be obvious that once a suit has been initiated, the psychiatrist risks even greater problems if he changes any material in the chart or even adds to the existing information.

There are relatively few lawyers who are sophisticated with regard to medical malpractice law and even fewer who know very much about the specialty of psychiatry. It is important that the psychiatrist's lawyer be as fully informed as possible as to standards of diagnosis and treatment which may be involved in a given case. It may even be useful to prepare a bibliography for the attorney which covers material relevant to the case.

Sometimes there may be disagreement between the doctor and the insurance company attorneys as to the desirability of settling a case out of court. A doctor may feel blameless and be inclined to fight a case to the bitter end in order to be vindicated. The insurers, however, may feel that litigating a case in court may be as costly as settling the case out of court, and may be even more costly if the case is lost. In past years policies were written so that the insurer could not agree to a settlement out of court without the doctor's consent. With the advent of so much malpractice litigation, however, some insurers have adopted a firmer stance. Some policies are now written so that the insurer can settle a claim without the doctor's consent. The doctor's opinion in this matter is taken seriously and may have considerable influence, but the attorneys representing the insurance company have the final say.

From a psychological standpoint, the most adaptive response to a lawsuit is to "stay cool." The natural reaction of the physician to a suit, particularly if it is viewed as unjustified, is fear and indignation. Although I have previously noted the substantial stress of a lawsuit, it is also true that the physician's fears as to the consequences of a suit are usually exaggerated. In one recent study of claims against psychiatrists, over half were dropped before any legal action was taken. Only 25% involved some legal process, 19% were settled by dollar payments, and 6% ended up in the courts.[17] The majority of lawsuits initiated against the psychiatrist do not end up in court, and only 20% of these end up with a favorable award for the plaintiff. The size of actual awards made against psychiatrists is not usually very high and the amount is most often covered by the doctor's insurance. Publicity is involved rarely in the average case, unless, of course, the incident involves moral misconduct such as sexual exploitation of a patient. Even if a suit is heavily publicized, the psychiatrist can usually rely on the empathy and support of most of his colleagues and patients. A highly publicized lawsuit obviously will hurt the psychiatrist's career, but it is unlikely to be catastrophic. Most psychiatrists who have been sued continue to practice successfully. Finally, the psychiatrist can at times gain comfort from the knowledge that in litigation which might involve the psychiatric profession as a whole, aid in legal defense can be obtained through the auspices of the Legal Action Commission of the American Psychiatric Association.

When litigation is pending, indignation accompanied by anger are responses which should be indulged only in private. "Blowing off steam" in front of colleagues or friends may make the psychiatrist feel better, but there is a slight danger that what is said may get back to the plaintiff or his attorney and be used to support their suit. The psychiatrist should exercise caution in deciding with whom he should ventilate his feelings.

Sometimes the clinician can gain a useful perspective by using his

---

[17]Slawson, "Psychiatric Malpractice: The California Experience," p. 141.

clinical skills and trying to understand what the plaintiff is experiencing. It may even be useful to try to go through the exercise of viewing the activities of the plaintiff as manifestations of an emotional disorder. To the extent that the plaintiff's behavior can be viewed as irrational, the psychiatrist's anger may be tempered and his wounded narcissism assuaged. It should be clear that I am recommending the adoption of a clinical view toward some aspects of the legal proceedings only as a means of promoting the psychiatrist's mental health. When it actually comes to dealing with litigation, the psychiatrist is advised to adhere scrupulously to the reality principle. This means looking after his own best interests and encouraging his attorney to be as aggressive as is necessary in defending the case.

What Legal Procedures Must a Psychiatrist Anticipate in a Malpractice Case?

The psychiatrist first becomes aware of the malpractice suit when he receives a summons and complaint. The summons is a document which names the parties to the lawsuit: the plaintiff or the party bringing the suit, the defendants and codefendants. It names the county in which the suit has been brought and the name of the plaintiff's attorney. The complaint is a document filed by the plaintiff which sets forth the facts of the problem which he alleges results from the defendant's malpractice. It asks for monetary damages and may list the amount of damages demanded.

The defendant physician has a limited amount of time in which to respond to the summons and complaint. He does have the option to file a motion called a demurrer to have the case dismissed on the grounds that it does not have legal validity. If he does not file a demurrer, or if he does and if the case is not dismissed, the physician defendant will respond to the complaint with what is called an "answer." In the answer, the physician responds to the patient's claims by denying allegations of negligence and admitting to whatever facts of the case may be true.

At this point in most states each party may exercise the right to elicit information from the other. Either party may submit to the adversary a list of questions to be answered under oath which are called written interrogatories. Either party may be questioned orally by the other's attorney and the oral testimony obtained is referred to as a deposition. Interrogatories and depositions are questions and answers similar to testimony in a trial, but they do not have the same influence as testimony which the jury actually obtains from a witness they can see and hear.

Once all the above information is prepared, the judge is likely to call a pretrial conference and attempt to settle the matter without a trial. If the parties do not agree to settle without a trial, the case is called and a jury is selected. In the actual trial each side begins by presenting its opening statement, which is a narrative account of what it expects its evidence to establish. Then the plaintiff presents his evidence. Usually, expert witnesses are called who are asked questions by the plaintiff's attorney in a process termed direct examination. The defendant's attorney then cross-examines the plaintiff's witness to try to discredit or confuse his testimony. Once the plaintiff's case has been presented the defendant can move for a directed verdict, which is really a motion asking the court to rule that the plaintiff has no case and that the suit should be dismissed. If this motion is denied, the defendant presents his case and the defendant's witnesses (which may include himself) are examined and cross-examined. The plaintiff then has the opportunity to present other evidence to rebut that given by the defendant. At this point the defendant can again move for a directed verdict. If this is denied, each side has an opportunity to present closing arguments to the jury. The judge then instructs the jury on the law, after which the jury deliberates and returns a verdict. Most states require unanimous verdicts to establish liability.

After the verdict is given, the side which has lost may decide to appeal. This usually leads both sides to present lengthy written and oral arguments to an appellate court. The plaintiff and the physician defendant do not have to be present at the appellate hearing. They do, however, have to be present at the actual trial, and indeed the physician is at a considerable disadvantage if he is not.

The above description of the litigation process is extremely oversimplified. Even this capsule account, however, may present some sense of how complicated and time-consuming a malpractice suit may be. There is currently great concern among attorneys, physicians, insurance companies, and the general public as to the costliness of this process. Many states now provide screening panels which examine cases before they get to the litigation process. These panels tend to discourage the pressing of weak cases and to encourage quick out-of-court settlement of strong cases. Other remedies which have been considered include the creation of arbitration panels which have the power legally to settle disputes, and a form of "no fault" compensation in which plaintiffs might receive small awards for damages without trying the issue of whether the physician was negligent. There are serious practical and legal problems with both of the latter solutions and neither has generated much enthusiasm.

What Kind of Financial Damages Can Be Assessed against the Psychiatrist Who Is Successfully Sued?

Although most suits for damages are filed by the party who is actually injured, psychiatrists can be also sued by relatives of the patient in cases of wrongful death. Psychiatrists have been sued by relatives of patients who have killed themselves and by relatives of individuals (third parties) who have been killed by the psychiatrist's patient.

As a general rule a psychiatrist who loses a malpractice suit must pay compensatory damages. Compensatory damages are based on the principle that the plaintiff should be restored to his preinjury condition so far as it is possible to do so. The effort here is to "award as much money as would be likely to restore the patient to the state he would be in if no harm had occurred." Sometimes this is referred to as "making the man whole again." Compensatory damages include not only medical expenses and impairment of working capacity, but physical and mental suffering as well. Attorney's fees and the cost of litigation are not usually included.

In rare instances the psychiatrist must also be concerned with punitive damages. Punitive damages can be viewed as a civil fine paid to the plaintiff with the direct intention of punishing the defendant and deterring him and others from similar conduct in the future. Such damages are not as a rule awarded unless the defendant has acted from a wrongful motive or at least with gross or knowing indifference for the rights of others. They are usually based on an element of outrage on the part of the public similar to that involved in a crime. Punitive damages may not be covered by the psychiatrist's insurer.

What Standards of Proof Are Utilized in Malpractice Trials?

When a malpractice suit reaches the stage of trial and must be decided by a jury (a relatively rare event in psychiatric practice), the jury must be instructed as to what method or standard of proof will be utilized. Unlike the situation in criminal proceedings where proof of guilt must be "beyond a reasonable doubt," in tort proceedings proof usually rests on a "preponderance of evidence." This means that the party having the burden of proving certain facts must make it appear more probable than not that those facts existed. The current standard of proof makes it difficult to predict the outcome of tort litigation and ensures that there will be many equivocal decisions. A 51–49% ratio of certainty on the part of the jury will have the same effect on the participants as a 99–1% ratio.

2

Intentional Torts in Psychiatric Practice

In the common law, wrongs which are inflicted intentionally are actionable. The element of intent is present when the wrongdoer is either motivated to harm another or realizes that a certain (usually harmful) result is substantially sure to follow from his actions. Some acts are both intentional torts and crimes and in these cases both civil tort action and criminal prosecution may be brought for the same wrongful conduct.

Although most medical malpractice involves allegations of negligence, patients also sue doctors who harm them through deliberate or intentional acts. In cases involving accusation of an intentional tort, expert testimony is not required to establish the liability of the defendant. This is different from the usual practice when a malpractice suit is based on negligence. Another important fact which psychiatrists must know about intentional torts is that they are not always included in the coverage provided by standard malpractice insurance policies. Psychiatrists should be especially careful in checking their policies and should be knowledgeable as to which wrongful acts on their part may not be covered.

Obviously the physician, just like any other person, can intentionally harm another individual. The inherent risk of committing an intentional harm, however, is not great in most aspects of medical practice. In psychiatry the situation is somewhat different. The practice of psychiatry often requires retraining patients and depriving them of freedom. In carrying out these tasks, there is some risk of committing battery or false imprisonment. The intimate nature of the psychiatrist–patient relationship is influenced by the consequences of physical touching, and some forms of touching with sexual intentions may be actionable. The material which the psychiatric patient discusses with the doctor is likely

25

to be more sensitive than that of other patients. Psychiatrists must be aware of the risk of suits for breach of confidentiality, invasion of privacy, and defamation. The close nature of the psychiatrist–patient relationship may also increase the risk that the psychiatrist might exert undue influence on the patient or defraud him.

There is some inconsistency as to whether cases involving some torts such as battery are tried under intentional tort or negligence theory. Such inconsistency may be determined by complicated legal theories, but it is also related to practical issues such as the statute of limitations (the time by law in which a suit must be instituted following an alleged wrong) being different for intentional versus negligent action and the availability of expert witnesses. When expert witnesses are not available, it may be to the plaintiff's advantage to try a case under an intentional tort theory (providing the physician is insured for that tort or is wealthy enough to pay the damages).

When May a Psychiatrist Be Sued for Assault and Battery?

Battery is a wrongful, harmful, or offensive contact with another's body which is intentional. An assault is quite similar to a battery except that the offending action may be one that puts the other person in fear of offensive contact. In both assault and battery, the defendant must have intended the offensive result or must have realized that the result was substantially certain to follow from his action. Although doctors are almost never sued for assault, they can be sued for battery. As a rule medical malpractice suits brought on the doctrine of battery are based on the physician's failure to obtain consent to perform a procedure. The "intentional" nature of the act in a battery action may not include intent to harm. It is only the content of the act which must be intended. The doctor may actually have quite benevolent motivations. A doctor may, for example, perform a procedure without telling the patient he is going to do so; or he may treat a young child who is incapable of understanding the nature of that treatment without the consent of the child's parents; or the doctor may obtain consent to do one type of operation, but do another.

In this type of tort the issue is not whether the doctor provided the patient with sufficient information to meet the requirements of informed consent. The issue is that the doctor obtained no consent at all.[1] Battery suits are usually argued under theories of intentional misconduct,

[1]A. R. Holder, *Medical Malpractice Law* (New York: Wiley, 1975).

whereas suits involving the doctrine of informed consent are usually tried under the theory of negligence.

In both psychiatric and nonpsychiatric medical practice it is often tempting to assume that patients who refuse physical examinations or medical and surgical interventions are incompetent and can be treated even if they protest. Too frequently, doctors are likely to impose treatment on the protesting patient when the patient has not been adjudicated incompetent. Nonpsychiatrists are especially cavalier in treating protesting patients who are assumed to have brain syndromes. This puts the doctor in jeopardy of a lawsuit for battery. In discussing patients who have not been adjudicated incompetent, one eminent authority notes, "The general rule is clear: patients may refuse to permit any medical or surgical procedure from being performed on them regardless of the opinions of the doctors as to the advisability of the treatment. The rule applies both in and out of the hospital."[2] Even a patient who is committed involuntarily may have a right to refuse treatment, and in some instances can sue for unwanted treatment. In one well-known case, a committed patient who had a religious objection to treatment was forcibly given major tranquilizers. The court held that the only circumstances under which compulsory medication may be given over the religious objection of the patient is if the patient has been behaving in a way that is harmful to himself or others. The court further held that in this case these conditions were not met.[3] In the state of Massachusetts, a civil rights action which includes a plea for damages against the psychiatric staff of a mental hospital has recently been made by civilly committed patients who were treated against their will.[4] In other states, psychiatrists are being advised to be cautious in forcibly treating patients who refuse treatment even if these patients have been committed. The problem of dealing with the patient's right to refuse treatment will be discussed in more detail in the second part of this book. Here, I will simply emphasize that the psychiatrist should not as a rule attempt to examine or treat a competent, nonconsenting patient whose behavior poses no serious threat to himself or others.

Psychiatric hospitals are liable for battery when patients are physcially abused by attendants or other employees. Successful actions against hospitals for assault and battery on the part of attendants have occurred.[5] It is also not unheard of for a physician to become involved in

---

[2]G. L. Annas, *The Rights of Hospital Patients* (New York: Avon Books, 1975).
[3]Winters v. Miller, 446 F.2d 65 (2d Cir. 1971).
[4]Rogers V. Okin, "Right to Refuse Drugs on Trial in Boston," *Psychiatric News 13*, no. 17 (1978): 1.
[5]Davis v. New York, 332 N.Y.S.2d 569 (N.Y. 1972).

efforts to restrain a patient in a manner that is excessively forceful.[6] In such cases the physician as well as the hospital can be sued for assault and battery.

Controversial therapies involving physical contact which inflict pain upon patients may also result in lawsuits. The most famous of these suits have been tried under a negligence theory, but the actions involved could easily have been construed as battery. The most frequently cited case involved a psychoanalyst who used a number of techniques involving physical contact such as wrestling with severely disturbed patients. The court held that the psychiatrist had beaten the patient on a number of occasions, that the psychiatrist's actions were intrinsically negligent, and that the plaintiff did not have to produce expert testimony in order to recover damages.[7] In another instance, a young woman undergoing rage reduction or Z-therapy, a form of treatment in which the patient is restrained, tickled, and poked while being questioned by the therapist, was awarded extensive damages for ensuing psychological harm, bruising, and acute renal failure.[8]

Battery is a crime as well as a tort. In cases where physicians have had forceful or fraudulent sexual intercourse with patients, they have been subject to heavy criminal penalties. Forcible rape or rape by fraud is, of course, rare in psychiatric practice.

Under What Circumstances Can a Psychiatrist Be Sued for Fraud?

In legal terminology, fraud is "an intentional perversion of truth for the purpose of inducing another who relies upon such misrepresentation to part with some valuable thing belonging to him or to surrender a legal right." It is rare for a psychiatrist or any other physician to be sued for fraud. There are, however, several situations in which such a suit might occur. A physician may totally misrepresent the risks of a given procedure to a patient, assuring the patient that there is little chance of serious harm when in actuality the procedure is dangerous. A psychiatrist who assured a patient that there was absolutely no risk to neuroleptic therapy or electroconvulsive therapy would in theory be liable for fraud. Another situation in which the physician may be liable occurs when he misrepresents the nature of a procedure which has been performed on a patient. Such a situation could arise if a psychiatrist were to prepare a patient for electroconvulsive therapy, fail to provide the

---

[6]Bellandi v. Park Sanitarium Association, 6 P.2d 508 (Cal. 1931).
[7]Hammer v. Rosen, 165 N.E.2d 756 (N.Y. 1960).
[8]Abraham v. Zaslow, #245862 Sup. Ct. Santa Clara Co., Cal., Oct. 26, 1970.

treatment, but inform the patient that treatment had been given. The possibility of such behavior on the part of a psychiatrist is, of course, remote. Placebo therapy, although certainly an intentional perversion of truth, is not a fraudulent action since it is designed to help the patient and is not initiated with the intent of inducing the patient to part with some valuable thing or to surrender a legal right.

Fraud can also occur when the physician knows that a treatment would have no reasonable medical justification but tells the patient that it is necessary, in the expectation of receiving a substantial fee. The key issue here is the intent of the physician. An expensive and unneeded treatment may be prescribed primarily because of the honest, if misguided, belief of the physician that it will be helpful to the patient. On the other hand, the prescription may be motivated by the physician's greed. There is usually no certain way of knowing what the intent of the physician was. In dealing with psychiatric patients, there is so much commitment to ideology and so many different justifications for all schools of therapy that the therapist can usually rationalize the necessity of a given treatment to himself or to others. Thus, we are unlikely to see suits for fraud in situations where psychoanalysis is recommended to a healthy person or where electroconvulsive therapy is given to a patient with a mild neurosis.

Willfully concealing negligence may also leave the physician liable for fraud. A psychiatrist may be tempted to keep his patient from finding out that a mistake has been made, but is always unwise to conceal facts. As a general rule, the adverse consequences of negligent practice are not nearly as drastic as the adverse consequences of a detected "cover-up." Patients who are harmed by treatment or who may be injured while hospitalized should be acquainted with the facts of the harmful incident. Details as to factors which may have produced the harm should be dutifully recorded in the patient's chart.

Psychiatrists often minimize the adverse consequences of biological therapies even after these consequences have already appeared. This is not fraudulent if the physician's intent is benevolent. A psychiatrist who tries to reassure a patient that the confusion following electroconvulsive treatment is a transitory phenomenon which is likely to disappear quickly may sometimes be incorrect. He is not, however, covering anything up, but is just trying to comfort the patient and diminish useless and complicating anxiety. The psychiatrist who de-emphasizes the patient's preoccupation with the side effects of psychotropic drugs is usually trying to diminish reinforcement of drug-created symptoms. His intent is to help the patient. The psychiatrist is not behaving fraudulently unless he is minimizing adverse consequences for his own rather than the patient's benefit.

The fraudulent behavior of physicians is sometimes treated as a crime rather than as a tort. Recently there has been much publicity concerning Medicaid fraud among psychiatrists as well as other physicians. Towery and Sharfstein note ten possible fraudulent practices with regard to third-party payment which may be relevant to psychiatry. These are: (1) billing for services more expensive than those actually provided; (2) billing for services not rendered; (3) billing for multiple services for members of the same family in the same day; (4) multiple referral between practitioners when there is no real necessity for services; (5) charging for physician's services actually provided by professionals not eligible for reimbursement; (6) offering or receiving kickbacks; (7) billing more than one third party for the same service; (8) distributing drugs indiscriminately to anyone who can pay; (9) making excessive profits from a legitimate treatment; and (10) directing patients to a particular pharmacy.[9]

Towery and Sharfstein point out that there are many instances in which actions of psychiatrists that fall under the above-listed practices may not actually conflict with standard practices, and that it is not always easy to determine when the psychiatrist behaves fraudulently. They note, however, that psychiatry as a profession is not immune to fraudulent practices and that there is an urgent need for the profession itself to define precisely what practices might be fraudulent.

What Malpractice Risks Are Involved in Violating the Patient's Confidence?

The issue of confidentiality is complex enough, and controlled by so many different ethical and social as well as legal factors, that many of its ramifications will be considered in a separate chapter. The focus here is restricted to malpractice, or the manner in which the psychiatrist can be sued for revealing confidences entrusted to him in the course of practice.

There is general agreement among all writers in the medical malpractice field that confidentiality is an important right of a patient and that the physician is obligated not to breach the patient's confidences. There is complete agreement that confidentiality is even more important in psychiatric practice. Texts on malpractice and forensic medicine repeatedly caution the doctor to avoid tortious disclosure of confidential information and imply that if the doctor is careless, suits are sure to

---

[9]O. B. Towery and S. S. Sharfstein, "Fraud and Abuse in Psychiatric Practice," *Am. J. Psychiatry 135*, no. 1 (1978): 92–94.

follow.[10] In actual practice, however, successful suits for disclosure of confidential information are rare. As recently as 1975, an eminent legal authority on malpractice stated, "While much lip service is paid to this type of lawsuit, no American appellate case has been found in which the patient has been able to recover money damages from the doctor due to an alleged breach of confidentiality."[11] This is a startling statement in view of the intense preoccupation of doctors and attorneys with this issue. In 1978 the New York Supreme Court awarded $20,000 in damages to a patient whose history of psychiatric treatment formed the basis of a book written by a psychiatrist and the psychiatrist's psychologist husband.[12] The plaintiff had sued for breach of confidentiality and invasion of privacy. This case represents the only appellate decision in which major damages have been awarded for violating the patient's confidences. It was an unusual case insofar as the patient's sexual fantasies, infantile memories, passions of hate and love, and intimate relationships with others were discussed in book form. It is unlikely that we will see a similar type of case in the near future.

One reason for the infrequency of suits involving breach of confidentiality is that most doctors, and especially psychiatrists, are very careful in protecting the patient's confidences. The ethical case for confidentiality and the need to preserve confidentiality in order to conduct psychotherapy have been inculcated in us from the beginning of our training. Another reason why suits regarding confidentiality are infrequent is that there are some situations in which the physician is given the legal privilege to disclose material about patients without fearing liability. (The physician's privilege to disclose should not be confused with "testimonial privilege," which refers to an evidentiary rule usually codified in a statute which limits the extent to which a physician can be examined in court about confidential information acquired during treatment. "Testimonial privilege" limits disclosure and the physician's privilege to disclose increases it.) When acting as an agent of the court, the physician is usually not liable for statements made to legal agencies. Psychiatrists are not liable for revealing the patient's confidences during commitment hearings. When the court orders the psychiatrist to testify, the psychiatrist is also protected from liability. Some statutes insulate the physician from liability for certain types of disclosures. A psychia-

---

[10]L. R. Tancredi, J. Lieb, and A. E. Slaby, *Legal Issues in Psychiatric Care* (Hagerstown, Md.: Harper and Row, 1975); D. J. Dawidoff, *The Malpractice of Psychiatrists* (Springfield, Ill.: Charles C. Thomas, 1973).

[11]Annas, *Rights of Hospital Patients*, p. 123.

[12]C. R. Leland, "Psychiatrist Encounters Perils in Publication," *Legal Aspects of Medical Practice* 6, no. 4 (1978): 51–53.

trist can never be sued for breach of confidentiality for reporting child abuse. Some provisions also confer a privilege on physicians to provide pertinent information to Professional Standards Review Organizations (PSROs). [13]

Even if suits in this area are rare, it is wise for psychiatrists to continue to be cautious in preserving confidentiality. Some violations of confidentiality would appear to be clearly actionable. The psychiatrist who gossips about a patient and uses the patient's name is obviously behaving foolishly. Even when the psychiatrist believes the identity of the person about whom he gossips is well hidden, there is a risk that others may identify the patient. The homily that "this is a small world" takes on an intense meaning for the psychiatrist who finds that his cocktail party comments have been retold to his patient.

Aside from situations in which there is a statutory obligation for the physician to disclose information (for example, when the patient has a contagious disease, when the physician suspects that the patient is abusing a child, or when the patient clearly indicates that he is going to kill a certain person), a physician should always be cautious in discussing his patient's business with any third party. Until this decade there were no successful lawsuits recorded against doctors who revealed adverse information to employers, insurance companies, or physicians in good faith. In a 1973 case, an Alabama court held that a physician who discloses confidential information to an employer without the patient's consent may be found liable for the harm resulting from the patient's loss of a job. [14] As a general rule, communications regarding patients made to insurance companies or potential employers should never be made without the patient's consent. Even communications to other physicians regarding the patient are better not made without the patient's agreement since the physician may be in a position to influence the patient's insurability or employability. (These issues will be expanded upon in a later chapter.)

A more controversial issue is whether the physician can be liable for disclosing confidential information to a patient's spouse. One danger here is that the psychiatrist can reveal certain kinds of information to the spouse which will be used against the patient in a future action to dissolve the marriage or in a battle for custody of children. Even if the marriage continues, information gained from the psychiatrist can be used to harass, intimidate, or persecute the patient. While there have

---

[13]S. H. King, "In Search of a Standard of Care for the Medical Profession," *Vanderbilt Law Review 28* (1975): 1266–75.

[14]A. H. Bernstein, "Unauthorized Disclosure of Confidential Information," *Hospitals 48*, no. 21 (1974): 126–35.

been a number of attempts to sue psychiatrists for divulging information to spouses, none has thus far resulted in damages against the doctor. This situation may change because there are different precedents in other English-speaking countries.[15] The American Medical Association has argued that reporting information about the medical condition of the patient to the spouse is not a breach of confidentiality.[16] My own view is that while a psychiatrist may not always risk incurring liability by sharing information with the patient's spouse, in the majority of instances such sharing represents unwise and sometimes unethical clinical practice. It is usually useful before treatment is instituted to have a clear understanding with the patient as to the exact conditions under which the doctor will communicate with the spouse and what kind of material will be shared. The consent of the patient would seem to be necessary before any breach of the therapeutic contract is made.

In dealing with outpatients who are not highly disturbed, the psychiatrist will sometimes encounter patients who do not want spouses or other relatives to know about the fact of their receiving treatment. If the patient is an adult, the psychiatrist can go ahead with treatment and accede to this request. Some psychiatrists more committed to family therapy might not want to be restricted by such conditions and would refer the patient to another therapist. But the psychiatrist would probably be in some jeopardy of breach of confidentiality if he treated the patient and ignored the patient's request to keep others from knowing that such treatment was taking place.

When the patient is hospitalized or seriously disturbed, the situation is somewhat different. There are reasons why spouses or close relatives might need to know of the serious plight of their loved one. Family members may be needed to participate in the treatment process or to make decisions regarding the patient's legal status. Or the patient may not be competent to make treatment decisions. In dealing with late adolescents who have reached maturity but who are still being supported by their parents, the psychiatrist will certainly risk parental anger if he fails to inform them that their child is very ill or hospitalized. Children of an elderly parent might be similarly offended if the doctor did not tell them about their parent's serious illness. While the law in this area is unclear and varies from state to state, prudence, decency, and good practice usually favor the psychiatrist's informing next of kin about the serious illness of a patient even when the patient objects to such disclosure.

[15]"Furniss v. Fitchett," *New Zealand Law Review 396* (1958): 904.
[16]A. R. Holder, "Disclosure of Confidential Information," *Journal of the American Medical Association 385* (1971): 216.

The intentional torts of invasion of privacy and defamation of character are intimately related to the question of confidentiality. The right to privacy or "the right to be let alone" is established in most states either by court decision or by statute, and has been recognized by the Supreme Court as a constitutional right. Invasions of privacy in the medical setting occur in two situations: (1) when there is an offensive intrusion upon the seclusion of another; or (2) where there is publicity of another's life which would be highly offensive to a reasonable person and not of legitimate concern to the public. In the latter situation it is difficult to distinguish invasion of privacy from breach of confidentiality. Suits are more likely to be brought under an invasion of privacy theory when there is extensive disclosure about the patient.

Lawsuits based on intrusion upon the seclusion of another in medical practice are usually based on the presence of nonessential persons during actual treatment. A physician who allows a third party who has no professional connection with the case to observe a medical procedure without the patient's consent is invading the patient's privacy. The risks of a suit are greatest if the treatment involves substantial physical exposure of the patient. In psychiatric practice it is not uncommon to allow students and other interested parties to participate in diagnostic and treatment conferences even though they have no professional involvement with the patient. When this is done without the patient's consent, the psychiatrist risks a lawsuit. It is prudent as well as ethical for the psychiatrist to obtain the patient's express consent in advance before individuals not directly involved in his care are permitted to see the patient being interviewed, or are in attendance at any conference relating to the patient's diagnosis or treatment.

The patient has an absolute right to refuse to participate in a teaching conference where he is on display before a large number of individuals who are not directly involved with his care.[17] The patient also has the right to refuse to see anyone not officially connected with the hospital or not directly involved in his care or treatment, and to refuse to see social workers and to forbid them from reviewing his records.[18]

Liability for publicity concerning a person's private life usually occurs in medical practice when pictures or information about the patient are published in medical journals without the patient's consent. Even with the patient's consent, the physician may be liable if the pictures or discussion are utilized for commercial purposes. The courts have been lenient toward physicians where pictures or discussion have tended to

---

[17]J. R. Waltz and F. E. Inbau, *Medical Jurisprudence* (New York: Macmillan, 1971).
[18]Annas, *Rights of Hospital Patients.*

serve a legitimate scientific purpose.[19] It is ethically and legally sound, however, for the physician to take all steps to disguise the identity of the patient. The question of what constitutes an adequate disguise is a serious and unresolved problem for psychiatrists who publish clinical case material. It is essential, of course, to delete names. Privacy can also be protected without distorting the writer's thesis by altering certain identifying characteristics such as the patient's sex, age, race, or occupation.

There are obvious limits to how much a case can be disguised and still be part of a scientific report. Many authors are reluctant to tamper with the authenticity of their case descriptions. Yet the details of a case, such as dreams or specific interpersonal relationships or specific activities, which may be so important from a scientific standpoint may also be so unique to a given individual that readers may be able to ascertain the identity of the patient. A significant number of people may know that the patient has been visiting the particular psychiatrist who has written the scientific paper. Conceivably these people could read the article, identify the patient, and learn something about the patient which would embarrass the patient or put him in a compromised position.

In my own writing I try to conceal the identities of patients discussed in as many ways as possible. When I present a case study or vignette, I try to ascertain that it will be altered in such a way that no parties other than those involved in the patient's care or the patients themselves might be able to determine the patient's identity. Holding the value of protecting the patient's privacy above the value of preserving the authenticity of a presented case makes sense when a writer like myself uses cases primarily to illustrate concepts. There are other situations, however, in which a case is unique and its presentation in the literature constitutes an original contribution. Disguising too many details in such situations is a disservice to medical science. Here the physician is wise to obtain the patient's consent to publish accurate information. Sometimes changing details which may not be relevant to the particular illness, such as geographical location or occupation, can be negotiated with the patient.

Defamation of character is a communication by one person about a second person to a third person in such terms as to diminish the reputation of the person about whom the discussion was held. The defamatory communication may be written or verbal. Publication or communication of defamatory matter in the form of written or printed words or pictures is called libel. Or libel may also be published by broadcasting or telecasting if the actor reads or follows a prepared script. The publication of

[19]Commonwealth v. Wiseman, 356 Mass. 251, 249 N.E.2d 610 (1969).

defamatory matter by spoken words or gestures is called slander. For a communication to be defamatory, it must tend to harm the reputation of another, to lower his esteem in his community, to cause persons to stop associating with him or dealing with him, or to expose him to scorn, ridicule, or contempt. Libel and slander may be actionable in some circumstances even when no special harm has been caused. The defamed person may not have to prove damage; it is presumed.

Physicians can defame character as easily as other people and obviously have many opportunities to communicate information which will diminish the reputation of patients. As a rule, however, the physician is well protected by the three major defenses to defamation: truth, consent, and privilege.

Some of the suits against psychiatrists on the grounds of defamation of character have actually involved situations in which the psychiatrist communicated accurate information about a patient to another party. (It would seem that these cases might more logically have been argued on theories of invasion of privacy or breach of confidentiality rather than defamation.) In these cases, the plaintiffs were unsuccessful.[20] Similarly, when a patient consents to have compromising facts revealed to a third party, there is no cause of action for defamation.

When the psychiatrist is examining a patient for the court and makes statements to the court or to attorneys, he is usually operating under a privilege to disclose information which prevents him from being sued for defamation. Public officials and others charged with the performance of public functions are similarly privileged. This protection holds even when untrue or malicious statements are made.

Psychiatrists can theoretically put themselves in jeopardy of a suit for defamation when their diagnoses are sloppy. Too often patients are written and spoken about as psychopathic, alcoholic, or psychotic when there is little evidence that this is true. Such inaccurate labeling published to a third party such as an employer or insurer may be considered a form of defamation even if the psychiatrist believes in the accuracy of his diagnosis. If the doctor was negligent or at fault in arriving at a diagnosis communicated to others, the belief in his own truthfulness may not protect him. The psychiatrist is in even greater jeopardy, of course, if he makes false statements about the patient without the patient's consent. Psychiatrists sometimes have an unfortunate tendency to talk about patients in diagnostic terms such as "psychopathic" or "paranoid" which have a pejorative quality. This is clearly unwise. We should also be careful in describing acquaintances or colleagues in insult-

---

[20]Berry v. Moench, 8 Utah 2d 191, 331 P.2d 814 (1958); Hammer v. Polsky, 36 Misc. 2d. 482, 233 N.Y.S.2d 110 (1962).

ing or diagnostic terms. It is a wonder that psychiatrists have not initiated more slander suits against one another for describing one another as incompetent or paranoid.

What Are the Liabilities of a Psychiatrist Who Intentionally Contributes to the Improper Restraint of a Patient?

There are a number of theories under which a psychiatrist can be sued for wrongfully restraining a patient. A psychiatrist may make a negligent examination of the patient and initiate a wrongful commitment even though he has no wrongful intention toward the patient. Such occurrences are extremely rare and are more appropriately considered under the heading of negligent diagnosis.[21] More commonly, malpractice actions related to the issue of involuntary commitment are brought under the doctrine of false imprisonment. This tort occurs when the plaintiff is confined to certain boundaries by the defendant and the plaintiff is mentally harmed by the awareness that he is not free to move about at will. When the psychiatrist is intentionally involved in an unjustified and inappropriate deprivation of the patient's freedom, damages against him are likely to be extremely high. Most of the cases in this area of law occurred before the 1970s in an era when legal protection of the patient in the civil commitment process was limited and the power of psychiatrists was largely unmonitored. There are a number of rather spectacular cases on record in which psychiatrists have acted with obvious malice and spite to help in the process of involuntarily hospitalizing certain individuals.[22] Psychiatrists have been known to initiate commitment for financial gain or to assist friends or relatives who wished to be rid of a troubling spouse. Psychiatrists have also been guilty of failing to comply with the statutory requirements of the commitment process, and in some instances have failed to examine the patient who is committed.[23] Even without proving malice, the fact of a psychiatrist's violation of statutory provisions providing for proper commitment of mental patients may be sufficient to make a case for false imprisonment. Obviously, the doctor who signs a commitment paper without having even examined the patient is in great danger of being sued for substantial damages.

In a recent case a doctor (not a psychiatrist) was successfully sued

[21]A. R. Holder, "Erroneous Commitment," *Journal of the American Medical Association 219*, no. 10 (1972): 1389.

[22]Stowers v. Wolodzko, 191 N.W.2d 355 (Mich. 1971); Maben v. Rankin, 358 P.2d 681 (Cal. 1961).

[23]Dunbar v. Greenlaw, 128 A.2d 218 (Maine 1956).

for an unjustified commitment not on grounds of false imprisonment, but on the grounds of abuse of process.[24] In this instance, a doctor went through all the required legal procedures in filling out the commitments papers to restrain a sixteen-year-old girl who wanted to leave a university and go home. The court ruled that since the patient had been hospitalized in compliance with legal procedures, there was no unlawful restraint of her freedom, but that such restraint was entirely unjustified on a medical basis. The court further ruled that her complaints supported an action for "abuse of process." The tort of abuse of process is defined as the use of a legal process against another to accomplish a purpose for which it is not designed. The court further felt that this particular commitment represented a perversion of the purpose of the commitment statute and thus constituted an abuse of process. This is an unusual case and is not likely to exert much influence on the practice of psychiatry. The doctor in this case went through the process of commitment without dealing with the content or criteria of commitment. He failed to present any evidence that the patient met the criteria for civil commitment which were operative in that state at that time.

It is important for psychiatrists to realize that aside from the rare possibility of being sued for negligent diagnosis, they must act maliciously, ignore the legal process, or deliberately abuse the process if they are to be sued for wrongful commitment. In spite of the admonition of so many attorneys that "prudence and caution" must be watchwords in the area of commitment, and in spite of the many threats of lawsuits which the doctor may hear from patients who are committed or about to be committed, the doctor is at no risk if he follows reasonable standards in conducting his examination, is not malicious, and sticks to the letter and spirit of the law.[25] All this is quite important to the young doctor in the emergency room who often worries excessively as to whether he will be sued for committing a patient. With current laws and practices it is extremely unlikely that a conscientious physician can be sued for initiating commitment. There are probably more legal risks to the emergency room or clinic physician who fails to initiate commitment. (But even these risks are minimal.)

Can a Psychiatrist Be Sued for Intentionally Exerting Undue Influence over a Patient?

Undue influence is wrongful persuasion which overpowers a person's will and causes him to do something that he would not have done

[24]Maniaci v. Marquette University, 184 N.W.2d 168 (Wisc. 1971).
[25]Application of Howe, 295 N.Y.S.2d 883 (N.Y. 1968).

of his own volition. The theory of undue influence has sometimes been invoked where therapists have had sexual relationships with patients. In such instances undue influence is an intentional tort which leaves the physician liable for damages.

More commonly, the physician is accused of undue influence when a patient sells the physician valuable goods or property at far less than market value or leaves the physician a large amount of money in a will. Litigation here is usually directed at voiding the contract or voiding the will. Damages are not usually sought against the doctor. If the patient or his heirs bring a charge of undue influence against the physician, the burden of proof is on the physician to show that such undue influence was not applied. This is often very difficult to do.

Psychiatrists who develop intimate relationships with their patients should obviously avoid becoming involved in business transactions with them. If for some reason the psychiatrist discovers he is going to be left a legacy in his patient's will, the psychiatrist should contact his attorney immediately for advice on this situation. There will usually be severe criticism toward a physician who is left a legacy in the will of any patient he has recently treated.

Is the Psychiatrist Liable for Infliction of Mental Stress upon His Patients?

There are no published cases in this area which deal with mental stress alone, but theoretically the psychiatrist who practices unorthodox techniques that put a great deal of stress on the patient could be liable for the tort of intentional infliction of mental stress. In the majority of cases involving negligent infliction of mental distress a successful suit is dependent on a requirement that the plaintiff's distress has produced a physical injury.[26] There is considerable disagreement as to just what constitutes a physical injury, but in the past, courts have been unwilling to redress psychic harm alone. Recently, in areas of tort law other than medical malpractice there has been considerable liberalization of the criteria for defining psychic damage. Psychiatrists who utilize high-stress-inducing techniques should be aware of such trends.

[26]Johnson v. Woman's Hospital, 527 S.W.2d 133, 138, 139 (Tenn. App. 1975).

3

The Theory of Negligent Malpractice

While intentional torts are probably of more concern to psychiatrists than to other physicians, the majority of malpractice cases in psychiatry as in other medical specialties are based on theories of negligence. Negligence implies fault on the part of the doctor. At the risk of being repetitious it must be reemphasized that the doctor is not liable simply because the patient suffered an untoward result in the course of treatment. Many patients do not respond favorably to treatment: some do not change, others experience deterioration of their conditions during treatment, and still others are made worse by the treatment. It would be impossible to practice medicine if the doctor could be sued every time there was a bad result. Aside from being liable for intentional wrongs, the doctor can only be sued when he has practiced negligently.

What Is Negligence in Medical Practice, and How Must Negligence Be Proven in a Malpractice Suit?

Negligence is conduct which falls below the standards established by law for the protection of others against unreasonable risk or harm. A key word in this definition is "conduct." It is what the doctor actually does that is important. Unlike the situation with regard to intentional torts, the motive and intent of the physician have little relevance. If through his conduct a physician creates an unreasonable risk of harm, he may be held negligent even though his actual subjective intent or motivation was to provide maximum health care to the patient. Negligence is the most important concept or principle in the area of tort liability. As a general rule all persons are under a duty to conduct themselves in all of their diverse activities so as not to create unreasonable harm or risk to others. (Negligence in medical practice is only one aspect of negligent conduct which can lead to court action and liability. Much of our current negligence law is directed toward dealing with injuries caused by vehicles.)

There are four components of the cause of action for negligent malpractice. In any suit the plaintiff must establish these components in order to recover damages. These components are:

1. There is a physician–patient relationship which creates a duty to the patient.
2. The duty is violated by the physician's failure to conform to required standards of care (that is, by the physician's negligence).
3. The patient is harmed or damaged.
4. There is a causal connection between the violation of the standard of care and the harm or injury.

How Is a Duty to the Patient Created?

The physician's duty to the patient arises out of the doctor–patient relationship. A physician–patient relationship can be viewed as a contractual arrangement. The physician may explicitly agree to perform certain treatments in exchange for a specific fee. At other times there is an implied contract. The exact details of the transaction are not spelled out, but the physician begins treatment with the consent of the patient and there is an expectation of compensation for the physician. Even though there is an explicit or implied contract in most physician–patient relationships, the duty of care demanded by the physician is imposed by society through tort law rather than through contract law. As long as the physician does not guarantee results, the usual physician–patient contract is viewed in malpractice law primarily as an acknowledgment that a duty has been created.

In dealing with unconscious patients or in situations where the physician may render services without promises or expectations of receiving a fee, there is no explicit or implied contract which creates a duty to the patient. Here a different theory of creation of duty applies. It is usually assumed that a physician who undertakes to render care to a patient creates a professional relationship with that person. Once the physician undertakes to render service, the physician–patient relationship exists even though there is no contract.[1] Where there is a

---

[1]Rule v. Cheeseman, 181 Kan. 957, 317 P.2d 742 (1957).

physician–patient relationship the physician owes a duty to the patient. It takes very little action on the part of the physician to create a physician–patient relationship and therefore to create a duty to the patient. The undertaking of even minimal service in the forms of discussing an illness on the phone, giving advice, or promising to see a patient, have been judged to be actions sufficient to establish a physician–patient relationship and a consequent duty.[2]

When the physician is functioning primarily as an evaluator and not as a treator of the patient, and is conducting the examination at the request of a third party, it is unlikely that liability will be imposed on the physician. As a rule physicians who do preemployment or insurance examinations are not viewed as having a duty to the patient and are not liable for negligence.[3] Physicians who examine defendants or plaintiffs at the request of the court are absolved of any risk of liability even if they negligently misdiagnose a condition. The court-appointed psychiatrist in a civil commitment case is also shielded from litigation. It should be clear, however, that there are instances in which the psychiatrist may become involved in initiating the commitment of a patient he has already been treating and to whom he owes a duty. Suits for negligent diagnosis are possible in this situation.

Third-party requests are often for treatment as well as evaluation. When parents ask a doctor to treat their child, the doctor owes a duty to the child. The situation is somewhat different when a doctor works for a company and is asked to treat employees of that company. Because of the old common law rule that an employer is not usually liable for injuries one employee causes another, the right to sue a company physician may be denied even if there is a doctor–patient relation.[4] If the company-employed physician is negligent, the patient's only remedy may be in Workmen's Compensation. Workmen's Compensation laws (which will be discussed in greater detail in Part III) provide a means of redress for accidents and diseases incurred in the course of labor. Common law doctrines make it extremely difficult to prove an employer's negligence. Workmen's Compensation laws set up boards which have more lenient standards for granting redress to employees. The amount of the awards under Workmen's Compensation is usually less than under malpractice law.

---

[2]O'Neill v. Montefiore Hospital, 11 A.D.2d 132, 135, 202 N.Y.S.2d 436, 439 (1960); Maltempo v. Cuthbery, 504 F.2d 355 (5th Cir. 1974).
[3]Batistella v. Society of the New York Hospital, 191 N.Y.S.2d 626 (N.Y. 1959).
[4]A. R. Holder, "The Physician as Fellow Servant," *Journal of the American Medical Association* 223, no. 10 (1973): 1203.

How Are Standards of Care Determined in Malpractice Suits?

The physician violates a duty to the patient by failing to practice according to standards of care. The determination of such standards is a complicated matter. In ordinary tort law the standard of conduct to which individuals are held is usually stated as "ordinary care," "due care," or "reasonable care" measured against the hypothetical conduct of a hypothetical person—"the reasonable man of ordinary prudence." The court asks what would the "reasonable man" have done under the same circumstances as those in which the defendant found himself. The conduct of the "reasonable man" defines standards of proper behavior. Physicians and other professionals obviously possess skills and knowledge in the practice of their profession that go beyond that of the ordinary person. The standards of conduct expected of them in their professional role will, therefore, be greater than those expected of the ordinary citizen, and the concept of the "reasonable man" must be modified. In malpractice law the "reasonable man" becomes the "duly careful member of the profession."[5] The standards by which this hypothetical person would practice become the standards which determine malpractice.

Because of the complicated nature of medical practice it is difficult for juries composed of laypersons to know what the conduct of a duly careful member of the profession would be. For this reason expert testimony or an acceptable substitute for it is usually required in determining standards of care. The only situations in which expert testimony might not be required would involve matters which are part of the common knowledge of any layman, cases involving informed consent where a lay standard may have already been adopted, and matters in which negligence may be inferred from the fact of an unexplained injury of the type that does not normally occur in the absence of negligence. These exceptions as they relate to psychiatry will be discussed later.

There are a number of important issues involved in defining standards of professional conduct through the use of expert testimony and there are variations in the manner in which these issues are handled in different jurisdictions. The following issues are especially critical.

1. Historically, professional standards have been articulated in terms of the customary or usual practice of members of the profession. The customary practice rule for determining standards focuses on the typical conduct of professionals. Such an approach to defining standards limits liability, particularly when

[5]A. R. Holder, *Medical Malpractice Law* (New York: Wiley, 1975), p. 41.

the rule defines the standard as it is utilized in a given geographical area. Customary practice in any given locality can be substandard. Because of a fear that a substandard custom in a local area might become immune to legal challenge, the courts are gradually beginning to reject the customary practice rule.[6] There is now a movement in the direction of redefining professional standards in terms of the accepted rather than the customary practice.[7] An accepted practice standard does not depend on historical or customary conduct. It is instead based on what a reasonable, competent member of the profession practicing in the same specialty as the defendant would be expected to do in order to conform to the approved professional practice.

2. The courts generally recognize that there are many competing schools of therapy and that a practitioner should not be penalized for following a course approved by at least a respectable segment of his profession. A physician does not incur liability by electing to pursue one of several recognized courses of treatment as long as that treatment is acceptable to a respectable minority of practitioners.[8] Unfortunately, the courts cannot adequately resolve the question of what constitutes a respectable minority. In a field like psychiatry where there are so many different and competing schools of treatment, the definition of a respectable minority is likely to be quite broad.

3. Several courts have enunciated that a medical professional who adheres to professional standards cannot be found negligent merely because he commits an error in judgment.[9] These rulings reaffirm the respectable minority rule and give the physician the right to choose among different therapeutic approaches even though his preference turns out to be wrong. They also emphasize the basic premise of fault-based liability, namely, that a physician will not be held liable merely because there is an unfavorable result from therapy. A judgment may be wrong, but as long as it was reasonable there is no liability. The key word is "reasonable." The physician must take reasonable and acceptable steps in arriving at his decision. If he makes his decision without benefit of data which could have been obtained by cer-

[6]Blair v. Eben, 461 S.W.2d 370, 373 (Ky. 1970); Darling v. Charleston Community Memorial Hospital, 33 2d 526, 211 N.E.2d 353 (Ill. 1965).
[7]J. H. King, "In Search of a Standard of Care for the Medical Profession: The 'Accepted Practice' Formula," *Vanderbilt Law Review 28* (1975): 1236–44.
[8]Chumbler v. McClure, 505 F.2d 489, 492 (6th Cir. 1974).
[9]Haase v. Garfinkel, 418 S.W.2d 108, 114 (Mo. 1967); Kortus v. Jensen, 237 2d 845 (Neb. 1976).

tain tests, his decision may be negligent rather than reasonable. The physician is protected from being liable for errors in judgment primarily in situations where he has been thorough in arriving at a diagnosis and initiating treatment, and where there is enough uncertainty as to which competing therapeutic techniques or diagnoses are most appropriate so that competent practitioners would have disagreed.

4. Some courts have tried to define standards in terms of the conduct of the average practitioner in the class to which the defendant belongs.[10] The current movement is away from the use of the word "average" in formulating standards. This makes sense because an "average" formulation could lead to the assumption that all physicians in America who fall below the mean are negligent in practicing medicine. If average is confused with median, half of our physicians would be negligent.

5. In past years practitioners were held to standards defined by the particular school to which they belonged. Apart from osteopaths and perhaps chiropracters, the same school standard has lost much of its practical significance. As a general rule these days nonmedical practitioners who undertake to treat medical disorders are held to standards of medical practice.[11] Psychologists, social workers, and nurses who become involved in providing treatments that can be defined as medical may be held to the standards of medical practitioners. If a physician undertakes procedures that are ordinarily carried out by a specialist, he may be held to a level of performance expected in that specialty. As a general rule, however, specialists are held to different and higher standards of care than nonspecialists, even where dealing with the same problem.[12]

The need to practice up to the level of a specialty is uniquely important to psychiatrists. In undertaking any psychiatric technique the psychiatrist must practice as a specialist. Many psychiatrists develop proficiency in one or two techniques such as psychoanalysis or family therapy and do not keep abreast of developments in other areas of psychiatry. When these practioners try to utilize pharmacotherapy or behavior therapy, they will be held to the same standards to which other psychiatrists who use these treatment modalities are held. The psychiatrist is wise

[10]Shier v. Freedman, 58 Wis. 2d 269, 206 N.W.2d 166 (1973).
[11]J. H. King, *The Law of Medical Malpractice in a Nutshell* (St. Paul, Minn.: West, 1977), p. 70.
[12]Simpson v. Davis, 219 Kan. 584, 547 P.2d 950 (1976).

to avoid treating patients with interventions he is not familiar with unless he is willing to call in a consultant or "brush up" on his knowledge of the use of such techniques.

6. Until quite recently the standard of care expected of a given doctor was determined by practice of other physicians in the same geographical area. The skill and knowledge of a physician were compared only to other physicians in the same geographical area on the theory that physicians practicing in isolated rural areas, for example, should not be expected to be as well trained and up to date as the physician in an urban area.[13] In our current era of great geographic mobility and easy access to information, these so-called locality rules are understandably being modified. The rural physician can now keep up with new medical developments almost as well as the urban physician. Even states which still apply the locality rule to general practitioners have held that specialists must adhere to national standards.[14]

7. Once professional standards have been defined on the basis of expert testimony there is still no assurance that the court will accept such standards. Most courts allow professional standards as determined by medical experts to establish standards of negligence. Other courts, however, have viewed professional testimony as to standards as only one form of evidence that due care has been provided.[15] These courts feel free to accept or reject such evidence in making decisions. Although there have been some well-publicized decisions in which the courts have failed to heed the standards established by experts, the trend in litigation has been toward greater reliance on expert testimony.

What Are Some General Obligations of the Physician Which Are Incorporated in Standards of Due Care?

There are certain types of expectations of due care which appear regularly in malpractice decisions. The physician is always expected to have adequate knowledge and skills and to use them with adequate diligence in dealing with a patient. While lack of diligence accounts for more lawsuits than lack of skills, negligence is not simply limited to carelessness. The physician who does not have the training to perform a procedure or to make a proper diagnosis may be negligent even if he is

---

[13]Incollingo v. Ewing, 282 A.2d 206 (Pa. 1971).
[14]Christy v. Saliterman, 179 N.W.2d 288 (Minn. 1970).
[15]Helling v. Carey, 83 Wash. 2d. 514, 519 P.2d 981 (1974).

extremely careful in his work.[16] Failing to consult a specialist when involved in clinical decisions which are beyond his skills can also get the physician in trouble.

One of the basic skills in psychiatry is the capacity to understand the patient's language and use of idiom. Effective diagnosis and treatment is difficult if not impossible without such skill. The psychiatric profession may be especially vulnerable to lawsuits in this regard since so many of its members (in some localities as many as 40%) are foreign medical graduates. Of course, many of these doctors have a superb command of the English language, but the majority are likely to encounter some problem in communicating with the patient. It is important that these psychiatrists concentrate on improving their language skills and not be hesitant to utilize colleagues freely as consultants when they are uncertain as to the quality of their communication with patients. Foreign residents whose language skills are marginal must be supervised very carefully when they assume responsibility for diagnostic or therapeutic procedures.

Many malpractice suits are decided against the defendant primarily because of the failure of the doctor to seek consultation. Asking for a consultation ascertains that expertise will be available to the patient in areas in which the doctor feels deficient. The request for a consultation is also evidence of the doctor's diligence. There is a point, of course, at which request for consultation can be abused and is nothing but an unnecessary expense for the patient. Excessive use of consultation is a form of defensive medicine, but it is certainly effective in avoiding malpractice suits.

The prudent physician should always inquire about previous treatment, and where possible should consult with the patient's former doctors. This is simply good practice and courteous behavior. Knowledge of previous treatment may influence decisions as to current treatment. Knowledge of results of previous tests may obviate the need to repeat expensive tests, and of course the patient's former doctor may know things the patient may not reveal to the new doctor which are highly relevant to the patient's health. Psychiatrists, perhaps more than other doctors, have a regrettable tendency to be somewhat cavalier in obtaining previous records and talking with the patient's former doctor. This is poor medical practice which increases the risk of being sued for malpractice.

Another general standard which is almost always imposed on the doctor is the need to keep abreast of current developments.[17] This is an

[16]Holder, *Medical Malpractice Law*, p. 43.
[17]*Ibid.*, p. 49.

extremely critical issue in all of medicine as new information develops at an accelerating rate. The rate of development of new knowledge in psychiatry may be somewhat less than in other specialties, but it is still necessary for the psychiatrist to keep up with new developments. This issue will become more important as we use more biological treatments and discover more serious complications of these treatments.

Finally, standards of due care usually emphasize the physician's obligation to follow up on his patient's progress. The doctor must be sure that the patient understands all of the instructions pertaining to use of medication, recreation or activities, and return visits. There is some question as to how much information regarding the effects of medications must routinely be given to patients. (This issue will be elaborated in a later section on informed consent.) But it should be absolutely clear that the patient must know that the use of some medications requires caution and sometimes restriction of certain activities. This is particularly relevant to psychiatry where many medications are prescribed which produce drowsiness.[18] Patients must be warned about drowsiness and how it may affect activities such as driving. If the patient gets into an accident and the physician has failed to warn him about drowsiness, the physician is liable for what are often heavy damages. The physician is obligated to try to ascertain that instructions are understood even when the patient does not have a good understanding of English.[19] Here it is useful to use a colleague or employee who speaks the patient's language as an interpreter.

How Can Standards of Care Be Developed When Experts Are Not Available?

Plaintiffs in medical malpractice suits often have difficulty in finding expert witnesses who will support their case. Members of the medical profession are usually reluctant to testify against one another. Lawyers and laypersons sometimes label this reluctance as a "conspiracy of silence."[20] More likely it is related to a distaste for court appearances, a wish to remain loyal to colleagues, and an honest (although probably erroneous) conviction that the majority of malpractice lawsuits are unjust or malicious.

Given the reluctance of doctors to be experts, attorneys have sought

---

[18]Kaiser v. Suburban Transportation System, 398 P.2d 14 (Wash. 1965); Whitfield v. Daniel Construction Co., 83 S.E.2d 410 (S.C. 1965).
[19]Krushilla v. United States, 287 F.2d 34 (CCA 2, 1961).
[20]King, *Law of Medical Malpractice*, p. 81.

ways of establishing standards of care without the aid of experts. The most frequently noted doctrine that might circumvent the need for expert testimony is the so-called "common knowledge doctrine." According to this rule, the alleged negligence of physicians may in some situations be comprehensible to laymen without the guidance of expert evidence. The common knowledge doctrine is applicable only to situations of gross negligence.[21] It has been invoked primarily in surgical practice where there has been obvious clumsiness or carelessness. Other than situations in which the psychiatrist is physically abusive to the patient, it is difficult to create plausible scenarios as to how the common knowledge doctrine might be invoked in negligence malpractice as it relates to psychiatry.[22]

Sometimes the physician defendant admits that he was negligent either in his depositions or in his testimony. Here, expert testimony is not needed to establish his liability. Recently, some courts have compelled the defendant physician to be a witness and to respond to the questions calling for an expert's opinion regarding the issue at hand.[23] Obviously, the physician's attorney will vigorously resist efforts by the plaintiff's attorneys to elicit admissions or to make use of admissions obtained in depositions.

In negligence cases related to drug misuse, efforts have been made to rely on the package insert or the *Physician's Desk Reference* to determine standards of practice. There have been cases where physicians have departed from the relatively explicit recommendations of the manufacturer and have been held liable for untoward results partly because these recommendations have been viewed as standards.[24] Usually, however, brochures and instructions relating to drug misuse are more likely to complement expert testimony regarding standards and are unlikely to substitute for expert testimony.

Similarly, medical journals and books have not supplanted the need for experts. Medical literature is generally considered hearsay and is not admissable as direct evidence to prove statements it contains.[25] There are exceptions in some states, however, and in federal rules of evidence medical treatises have some authority when the expert relies on them during direct examination or if their existence is properly called to his attention upon cross-examination. Some states may also allow the use of

[21]Hestbeck v. Hennepin County, 297 Minn. 419, 212 N.W.2d 361 (1973).
[22]S. Messinger, "Malpractice Suits—the Psychiatrist's Turn," *Journal of Legal Medicine 3* no. 21 (1975): 20–31.
[23]Robertson v. LaCroix, 543 P.2d 17 (Okl. 1975).
[24]Mulder v. Parke Davis and Co., 288 Minn. 332, 340, 181 N.W.2d 882, 887 (1970).
[25]*McCormick on Evidence*, 744 E. Clears, ed., 2d ed. (St. Paul, Minn.: West, 1972).

learned treatises to impeach an expert's testimony. There is a wish on the part of attorneys to have the use of learned treatises supplant the need for experts, and there has been some slow change in this direction, but in most courts the use of medical literature as a source of expertise is limited.

On the other hand standards or guidelines developed by professional organizations and institutions have had considerable influence in some cases. In a well-known psychiatric case, standards for electric shock treatment prepared by the American Psychiatric Association were not adhered to. These standards were admitted as evidence as the prevailing standard of care and a judgment was awarded to the plaintiff even though expert witnesses were not called.[26]

Violation of statutes or government regulations may also justify liability for negligence without expert witnesses. In a recent case a child sued a physician in a hospital for alleged negligence for failing to report abuse of the child. This failure allegedly resulted in further injury to the child. Since there was a statute which required reporting of any battered child, the court held that expert testimony was not mandatory to prove a duty on the part of one who diagnosed child abuse.[27] It is conceivable that with a greater governmental regulation of medical practice new rules may eventually come to be viewed as standards of practice which are in themselves sufficient and which supplant the need for expert testimony.

Sometimes the plaintiff may try to prove negligence indirectly on the basis of circumstantial evidence. This manner of establishing evidence is often referred to as the doctrine of *res ipsa loquitur* (translated literally, "the thing speaks for itself"). In these situations although direct evidence of the precise reason the injury occurred is lacking, the nature of the injury itself may so strongly suggest wrongful conduct that nothing more is necessary to allow the plaintiff to present the case to the jury. (A frequently noted example here would be that of a sponge or hemostat left in the abdomen following surgery.) There are usually three conditions to be satisfied for the doctrine of *res ipsa loquitor* to apply. First, the harm must be of a kind which ordinarily does not occur in the absence of someone's negligence. Second, it must be caused by an agency or instrumentality within the exclusive control of the defendant. Third, it must not have been due to any voluntary action or contribution on the part of the plaintiff.[28] The doctrine of *res ipsa loquitur* has limited rele-

---

[26]Stone v. Proctor, 131 S.E.2d 297 (N.C. 1963).

[27]Landers v. Flood, 131 Cal. Rptr. 69, 551 F.2d 389 (1976).

[28]A. R. Rosenberg and L. S. Goldsmith, *Malpractice Made Easy* (New York: Books for Industry, 1976), chap. 9.

vance for psychiatric malpractice. It has been invoked in cases involving suicide and harm following electroconvulsive therapy, but with little success.

What Are the Special Problems in Defining Standards of Due Care in Psychiatry?

Psychiatry is a controversial field in which it is almost impossible to speak of customary standards of care and in which there are continuing major disagreements over acceptable standards of care. Psychiatrists often disagree as to what conduct makes for a reasonably competent practitioner. There are so many different ways of treating similar conditions that the possibility of the psychiatrist's claiming an error in judgment (rather than negligence) is much greater than it would be in other branches of medicine. The profession of psychiatry has shown an unusual tolerance for the protection of minority viewpoints, almost all of which are granted a certain amount of credibility. In dealing with a profession in which patients with a similar diagnosis such as depression may be treated with psychosurgery, tricyclic therapy, monamine oxidase inhibitors (MAOI), lithium therapy, individual psychotherapy, group psychotherapy, or behavior modification, the court must often search in vain for a standard. Frustration with the vague standards of psychiatry accounts for some experts' anticipating a gradual move toward application of a contract rather than a tort theory of liability to psychiatric practice. A contract theory of liability would allow a remedy for a patient injured by a respectable, but totally ineffectual, therapy.

How Is Harm or Injury to the Patient Established?

As a rule the extent of damages or harm claimed by the plaintiff must be substantiated by expert testimony (unless, of course, the patient is deceased).[29] The degree of damage is a critical factor in determining the size of the plaintiff's award. In psychiatric practice when patients are physically harmed as a result of biological treatment (or in rare instances because of battery during controversial forms of psychotherapy), the extent of harm is relatively easy to determine. Deterioration in the patient's emotional state as a result of negligent treatment is more difficult to prove since it involves such difficult-to-define factors as demoralization, stigmatization, and harm to reputation. There is always the possibil-

[29]W. Prosser, *The Law of Torts*, 4th ed. (St. Paul, Minn.: West, 1977).

ity that the harm claimed actually existed before treatment was initiated. The courts are also wary of taking psychic injuries too seriously since there is a widespread belief that these deficits are easier to simulate than physical injuries.

How Is Causation Proven in Malpractice Suits?

The final element of negligence is proof of the causal connection between failure to adhere to professional standards of conduct and the harm experienced by the patient. Attorneys divide causation issues into two categories: first, cause in fact; and second, legal cause. Both must be established before liability may be imposed.[30]

Cause in fact is established by evidence that tends to show that the conduct of the physician was a necessary antecedent to the plaintiff's injury. Many courts express this in the form of a rule commonly known as the "but for" rule.[31] The physician's conduct could not have caused the injury if the injury would have occurred without it. The "but for" doctrine puts causality in a frame of reference that is familiar to physicians. In medical terminology, a physician's conduct may be a necessary but not a sufficient cause of an event.

Sometimes the test for causation is that the defendant's conduct has been a substantial factor in producing the injury. The substantial factor test is of some usefulness to the plaintiff when two or more factors may be involved in an injury and where either one alone may have been a substantial factor in the injury. In this situation the "but for" test strictly applied would deny recovery, but the more flexible substantial factor formula would allow recovery.[32]

The second element of causation, legal cause, is primarily a device for limiting the scope of liability to those consequences of the defendant's conduct which bear some reasonable relationship to the risk he created. Legal cause is also referred to as "proximate cause." The concept of proximate or legal cause deals less with the issue of causality as physicians are used to thinking about it than it does with the issue of fairness. It is a concept used to limit liability by requiring that there be a legal proximity in the sense of justice or fairness between negligent conduct and its consequences. Experts in tort law view proximate cause as an elusive concept, and some experts believe that the concept should not even be considered an issue of causality.[33]

[30]E. J. Kionka, *Torts in a Nutshell* (St. Paul, Minn.: West, 1977), p. 29.
[31]Speed v. State, 240 N.W.2d 901 (Iowa 1976).
[32]Restatement of Torts 2nd. *American Law Institute*, 1965.
[33]C. G. Post, *An Introduction to the Law* (Englewood Cliffs, N.J.: Prentice-Hall, 1963), p. 73.

The task of linking negligent conduct to injuries is especially difficult as applied to psychiatric practice. Psychiatry is at a primitive stage of developing an understanding of etiology. We can say very little about the necessary or sufficient causes of most of the disorders we treat. Since we are not always clear as to what the natural course or prognosis of a disorder may be, it is often difficult to determine when harm is related to the disease process and when it is related to treatment. It is also difficult to determine whether use of a given treatment (or too much treatment or too little treatment) is the cause of harm. All these judgments are especially difficult to make when the injuries for which causes are sought are likely to be psychic injuries, the existence and extent of which are difficult to prove.

4

Malpractice Issues Arising during Initial Contacts with the Psychiatric Patient

The psychiatrist who meets the patient for the first time in the office, the hospital, the emergency room, or some other setting is immediately subject to the regulation of both statutory and malpractice law. Statutes may require the psychiatrist to report gunshot wounds and child abuse, or they may prevent the physician from giving narcotic drugs to a person who is suspected of being an addict. Statutory law also governs the process of voluntary and involuntary commitment to a mental hospital. The psychiatrist who decides to hospitalize an adult or child must be aware of the procedural requirements of the law and follow them assiduously. Frequently, statutory and malpractice regulatory factors are intertwined. Failure to follow statutory regulations with regard to civil commitment, for example, may subject the psychiatrist to a malpractice action. The main emphasis in this chapter is on malpractice risks which arise when the psychiatrist–patient relationship is initiated and the psychiatrist assumes a duty to the patient. Statutory law will be noted only as far as it has implications for malpractice. Discussion of statutory regulation of psychiatry with particular emphasis on civil commitment will be discussed in detail in Part II.

Frequently, the psychiatrist–patient relationship is initiated in the emergency room. Because of recent trends in medical care delivery the emergency room has increasingly become a primary source of care for the surrounding community and especially for the poor.[1] Many patients

[1]E. C. Shortliffe, T. S. Hamilton, and E. H. Naroian, "The Emergency Room and the Changing Pattern of Medical Care," *New England Journal of Medicine 258* (1958): 20–25.

tend to use emergency rooms as primary health services at times when they cannot reach their private physicians. Some of the patients seen in the emergency room need urgent care and some do not. The physician has no choice but to assume that every patient is an emergency case until he has examined the patient and concluded otherwise. It is especially difficult to determine when a psychiatric patient needs emergency treatment since accurate diagnosis and treatment in psychiatry usually takes more time than in other branches of medicine.

At What Point Does a Psychiatrist Who Counsels a Friend, Acquaintance, or Employee Assume a Doctor–Patient Relationship with a Resulting Duty of Care?

There is no clear answer to this question. When a psychiatrist responds to a casual question outside of a situation in which a professional relationship would ordinarily be thought to exist there is certainly little likelihood that the courts would assume a duty of care. Questions asked of psychiatrists at cocktail parties or other social situations to which the psychiatrist responds out of simple politeness do not create a physician–patient relationship since the psychiatrist is clearly not accepting the person seeking advice as a patient.

The situation is more complicated, however, when one sits down and listens to the troubles of a friend, acquaintance, or employee and provides some kind of advice. Every psychiatrist has encountered situations where people he knows, including colleagues, have asked to talk over problems with him. As a rule it is difficult to avoid responding to these requests out of simple kindness, concern, or politeness. The prudent psychiatrist who responds to requests for counseling should clarify the nature of his relationship with the person counseled. He should note his willingness or unwillingness to be that person's doctor. If he does not want to assume a medical role, he should make it clear that he is acting as a nonprofessional listener. Failure to define a nonmedical role may lead to the psychiatrist's falling into an advice-giving role which might be defined as a doctor–patient relationship.

Many doctors, including psychiatrists, have an unfortunate habit of casually giving medications, often antianxiety drugs, to friends. A neighbor, for example, may report difficulty in sleeping and out of kindness the doctor may prescribe or give that person a small dose of a benzodiazepine. In giving or prescribing any kind of medication the doctor is very likely establishing a relationship with a patient and a duty of care. He may be subject to legal action if there are untoward responses to his mild intervention.[2] It should also be noted that in some states there are statutes which make it illegal to provide controlled substances to a patient unless a formal medical record is kept on a patient. Thus, no matter how minor the act of giving a pill to a friend or neighbor may seem, the physician is unwise to do so unless he is willing to accept that person as a patient and to treat him as he would any other patient.

A physician who promises to see a patient may have created a duty of care, particularly if the promise is made in a setting that suggests an implied agreement to perform services in exchange for a fee.[3] Even the physician who allows his name to be used to have a patient admitted to a hospital for emergency care may have created a duty of care.[4] Whenever the physician sees a patient and takes a history and renders any kind of advice or treatment, he has established a physician–patient relationship. This is true even if it is the first encounter between the doctor and the patient and holds irrespective of the setting in which the encounter occurs.

Can a Psychiatrist Refuse to Treat a Patient?

Unless working in an emergency room, any physician has the right to refuse to see or treat any patient. The so-called "no duty" rule protects the rights of any individual, including a physician, to say no.[5] It preserves the freedom of the physician in a free-enterprise society.

Like other physicians a psychiatrist can limit his practice, and where consistent with sound medical practice he can refuse to perform certain types of medical procedures. A biologically oriented psychiatrist may not want to provide psychotherapy. It is usually wise for a psychiatrist to make clear to the patient, preferably by phone or by a brief interview before the first diagnostic interview is even scheduled, as to any significant limitations on his practice. This is ethical and practical as well as legally useful. A psychiatrist who limits his practice to certain techniques will usually elect to send patients who need other modalities of therapy to another doctor. Patients can be spared the inconvenience and psychological discomfort of having to report their problems to a second doctor if they are warned beforehand as to how the first doctor limits his practice.

Often the psychiatrist sees a patient in the office or in the emer-

---

[2]A. R. Holder, *Medical Malpractice Law* (New York: Wiley, 1975), p. 4.
[3]Maltempo v. Cuthbert, 504 F.2d 325 (5th Cir. 1974).
[4]Giallanza v. Sands, 316 So. 2d 77 (Fla. 1975).
[5]Hurley v. Eddingfield, 59 N.E. 1058 (Ind. 1901).

gency room and after an examination decides that he does not wish to see that patient. Scheduling problems, personal characteristics of the patient, or monetary considerations may influence this decision. It should be clear in this type of situation that a physician–patient relationship has been created. The psychiatrist now has a legal as well as an ethical obligation to help the patient find another physician and must be available to the patient until the new doctor has been found. The physician who evaluates a patient and merely informs that patient that treatment will not be offered and does nothing more to help the patient find a new doctor is not behaving ethically and may be legally liable under the doctrine of abandonment.[6] (The issue of abandonment will be discussed in Chapter 6.)

What Are the Psychiatrist's Obligations if He Encounters an Accident?

The physician is never obligated to stop to render assistance when he encounters an accident. Many physicians claim they are afraid to stop at accidents because they fear malpractice suits. The fear is usually unrealistic. Almost all states have enacted "good samaritan laws" which are designed to eliminate recovery of damages for ordinary negligence in the course of medical treatment at the scene of an accident.[7] These laws vary from state to state, but in most situations they provide the doctor with relative freedom from liability. The doctor need not be licensed to practice in the particular state in which the accident is encountered. Nor is he obligated to continue to treat the victim once competent assistance has arrived.

Good samaritan laws vary widely in the degree of protection from liability offered to the physician. Most of them, for example, still may find the physician liable for "gross negligence."[8] A drunken physician who stops to render assistance that aggravates the patient's injury could be liable.

Even in states that do not have good samaritan laws the physician who stops to render assistance is not expected to perform as skillfully as he might in an emergency room or a medical clinic.[9] He is usually expected to perform with a degree of skill, care, and knowledge that the average practitioner would use under the circumstances imposed by the

---

[6]A. R. Holder, "Abandonment, Part I," *Journal of the American Medical Association* 225, no. 9 (1973): 1157.

[7]N. C. Chayet, *Legal Implications of Emergency Care* (New York: Appleton Century Crofts, 1960).

[8]Holder, *Medical Malpractice Law*, p. 9.

[9]*Ibid.*

emergency. An interesting question here is whether a psychiatrist, who often lacks skills in dealing with medical emergencies, would be held to the level of skill of an average practitioner of medicine or to the level of skill of a psychiatrist. This question is primarily of theoretical interest and there are no records of suits against psychiatrists who have rendered aid at accidents. The ethical psychiatrist should try to render assistance in an accident to the best of his ability. Even if he has not kept up his emergency medicine skills, he is likely to be more helpful than the average citizen and the risks of being sued are minimal.

Must a Hospital Render Service to Someone Who Comes to an Emergency Room for Psychiatric Treatment?

If an emergency is found to exist, the hospital with emergency facilities is required to render service. Emergencies have been legally defined as injuries or acute medical conditions liable to cause death or disability or serious illness. They include acute psychotic states and suicidal conditions.[10] It should be apparent that there is no way of knowing if a patient who appears in an emergency room and requests to see a psychiatrist is psychotic or suicidal. Until the psychiatrist has talked to such a patient, there is no way of knowing whether a psychiatric emergency exists. The psychiatrist working in the emergency room is at legal risk if he fails to evaluate any patient who appears for psychiatric assistance.

How Long Must a Patient Wait to Be Seen?

The patient must be seen in a reasonable time and there has been litigation if damages have occurred during the period of waiting. Presumably if a suicidal patient waited for hours to see a psychiatrist, became disheartened, and ran off and killed himself, the doctor and the hospital might be liable. The American College of Surgeons has recommended that medical staff coverage be sufficiently adequate so that a physician could see every patient fifteen minutes after arrival.[11] Some attorneys feel that this recommendation could be used as a standard. There would be considerable question in my mind whether such rapid service could conceivably be provided in a busy emergency room which sees many psychiatric patients.

[10]G. J. Annas, *The Rights of Hospital Patients* (New York: Avon Books, 1975).
[11]*Bulletin of the American College of Surgeons*, May–June 1963, p. 112.

Does the Patient Who Comes into an Emergency Room Have the Right to Be Seen by a Physician?

The answer to this is an unequivocal yes. Attorneys agree that only a physician can make a diagnosis of an emergency.[12] A physician who agrees to be on call must see the patient. It is not sufficient for a nurse or attendant to evaluate the emergency room patient. Nor is it sufficient for the doctor merely to talk on the telephone or to evaluate by telephone conversation the patient who has already arrived at the emergency room.

Once the Physician Initiates Treatment of an Emergency Room Patient, for How Long Must Treatment Be Continued?

A hospital with an emergency room must continue to provide service until the patient can safely be transferred to another hospital or can be discharged without harm. A psychiatrist cannot simply discharge a psychotic or suicidal patient who needs treatment and is willing to accept it. He must either hospitalize that patient or work out a satisfactory disposition which includes outpatient follow-up. In some situations the only recourse with a suicidal patient is hospitalization. Hospitals which have emergency rooms do not always have facilities for caring for disturbed psychiatric patients. Here the emergency room physician is confronted with the problem of transporting the patient to a suitable hospital, often in the middle of the night. The doctor has considerable responsibilities in this area. A patient may agree to go to another hospital but may lack the competence to get there without mishap. Such a patient should never be left to navigate on his own, but should be assisted by friends, family, hospital employees, or, if necessary, the police. If no help in transporting the patient can be obtained, the patient should be kept in the admitting hospital and treated as effectively as possible until safe transfer can be arranged.

Patients whom the physician believes are in need of continual emergency care, but who refuse it, are an especially trying problem. Depending on the statutes in effect in a particular state at a given time, the patient may have to be discharged against medical advice or civilly committed. If a petition for commitment has been made and the patient needs transportation to another hospital, the police must usually take him there.

[12]Z. Letourneav, "Legal Aspects of the Hospital Emergency Room," *Cleveland Law Review* 16 (1960): 50.

Is Emergency Room Treatment Ever Based on Prepayment or Demonstration of Ability to Pay?

Emergency rooms cannot turn away patients for financial reasons. Even the most poverty-stricken patient must be seen. Patients who might happen to have large outstanding bills at the hospital must also be seen.

Must the Patient's Physician or Psychiatrist Be Consulted before Emergency Room Treatment Can Begin?

The answer to this question is clearly no. It is both polite and useful for a psychiatrist to call a colleague and let him know that his patient has appeared in the emergency room. A conscientious psychiatrist would probably want to come down to the emergency room and treat the crisis situation himself. The emergency room doctor, however, has no legal obligation either to inform other doctors that their patient has appeared at the emergency room or to receive their permission to treat the patient.

Must an Inebriated Patient Who Is Behaving in an Obnoxious Manner Be Examined and Treated?

If an inebriated patient comes to the emergency room asking for help, he must be examined; and if he needs and accepts treatment, he must receive it.[13] If the patient is uncooperative in accepting treatment but still desperately needs it, efforts should be made to determine if the patient meets the criteria for involuntary commitment or incompetency or whatever procedures in a particular jurisdiction will allow for involuntary treatment. The considerations governing the doctor's actions would be similar to those discussed in Part II.

What Should Be Done with a Psychotic Patient Who Comes to the Emergency Room Asking for Help, but Who Refuses to Come into the Hospital and Refuses to Take Medication?

Treatment should never be imposed on a patient who actively refuses it unless the doctor is almost certain that failure to provide treat-

[13]W. A. Bellamy, "Malpractice Risks Confronting the Psychiatrist," *American Journal of Psychiatry 118*, (1962): 769–78.

ment will lead to the patient's death. In life-threatening situations the ethical doctor will usually treat the patient first and worry about legal considerations later. Psychiatrists are usually not faced with this problem since immediate lifesaving treatment is rarely needed in psychiatric emergencies.

Patients who are noncommunicative, who do not verbally consent to treatment, but who do not refuse or physically resist it may be viewed as consenting to treatment. If the patient refuses treatment but meets statutory criteria for involuntary commitment, a commitment petition should be instituted. In some jurisdictions this will allow for the initiation of treatment. In other states, however, even initiation of commitment may not give the doctor the right to proceed with treatment unless the patient is an immediate danger to himself or others. In these states an additional finding of incompetency may be required if the patient's refusal to accept treatment is to be overruled. When the physician has a clear conviction that a patient who needs treatment and refuses it is competent and not committable under the state's laws, the only recourse is to discharge the patient against medical advice. (The patient's right to refuse treatment, commitment laws, and incompetency proceedings will be discussed in Part II.)

If the Psychiatrist Believes That a Patient Seen in the Emergency Room Is Potentially Suicidal or Homicidal and the Patient Refuses Help or Hospitalization, Must the Psychiatrist Initiate Commitment Proceedings?

In most states psychiatrists may petition to commit a patient, but the law does not require them to do so. If someone else has already petitioned for the patient's commitment, the psychiatrist may of course be asked to examine the patient and state an opinion as to whether commitment is warranted. When functioning as an agent of the court the psychiatrist is not usually liable for a negligent diagnosis. The malpractice implications in this area are relevant primarily to those instances in which the psychiatrist is the petitioner. The emergency room psychiatrist may find himself in the petitioner role frequently. Highly disturbed patients may walk into the emergency room or be accompanied by family, friends, or police who subsequently disappear. The psychiatrist is then left with a severely disturbed patient who is resistant to treatment and hospitalization. In this situation the psychiatrist must either petition for commitment or allow the patient to leave.

There are no cases on record of a psychiatrist's being sued for failing to petition for commitment of a patient who subsequently hurts himself or someone else. Perhaps such suits have occurred, but neither the psychiatrists nor the attorneys with whom I have checked have heard of them. This is surprising because legal authorities frequently advise psychiatrists that they are obliged to petition for commitment when patients meet commitment criteria. Psychiatrists have certainly been held liable for releasing already hospitalized patients who subsequently injured themselves or others.[14] It would seem that psychiatrists could in theory be sued for failing to initiate the commitment of a patient who subsequently harms himself or others. One possible exploration of the absence of such suits is that psychiatrists are extremely cautious in dealing with dangerous patients and may protect themselves by liberal use of the commitment process. There is ample evidence that psychiatrists overpredict dangerousness to self or others. When in doubt, psychiatrists take the most conservative course and initiate commitment.

Another possible explanation is that the plaintiff would be unable to provide proof that the doctor was negligent in failing to diagnose the patient's dangerousness. As a rule only the emergency room physician and the patient know what transpired during the examination. If the physician has released the patient, he has probably written a note which documents his judgment that the patient was not dangerous. Even if the physician is proven wrong, in the absence of additional evidence he has only committed an error in judgment and is not liable.

What Issues Should the Psychiatrist Consider in Determining Whether or Not a Minor Can Be Treated without Parental Consent?

As a general rule parental consent for any form of medical treatment of a child is desirable. There are a number of situations in the practice of medicine, however, where such consent is not necessary or possible. There are special statutes, for example, which allow the child alone to consent to treatment for venereal disease and to receive contraceptive devices.[15] With the exception of very young girls, a physician is probably protected if he performs an abortion on a girl who refuses to tell her parents that she is pregnant.[16] Children can be treated in emergency situations without the parents' consent when the parents cannot be immediately reached.[17] Emancipated minors who are self-supporting or living away from home may independently consent to treatment.[18] It is not uncommon for adolescent patients to consult psychiatrists inde-

---

[14]*Ibid.*

[15]A. R. Holder, "Treating a Minor for Venereal Disease," *Journal of the American Medical Association 214*, no. 10 (1970): 1949.

[16]Jones v. Smith, 278 So. 2d 239 (Fla. 1973).

[17]Luka v. Lowrie, 136 N.W. 1106 (Mich. 1912).

[18]Bach v. Long Island Jewish Hospital, 267 N.Y.S.2d 289 (N.Y. 1966).

pendently and request treatment. Often they insist that their parents not know that they are receiving psychiatric help. The psychiatrist probably does not risk liability by agreeing to the conditions of confidentiality set by such patients, but it is usually unwise to continue treatment of the adolescent for any length of time without the parents' knowledge. A psychiatrist's services in this instance might not be compensated, and even if the patient's parents learned about the treatment later they would have a right to refuse to pay the bill. More important, in a majority of instances the child's wish to keep the parents uninformed about his being in therapy is based on irrational motivations. The maintenance of secrecy can by itself impair the therapeutic process. As a general rule therapy goes smoother if the parents know of its existence.

On occasion I have seen adolescent patients as young as sixteen who requested an appointment and did not reveal that their parents were uninformed that they had done so until the interview was under way. In such instances I have usually told the adolescent that I would not continue treatment unless his parents were at least aware that I was seeing him. I also assure the adolescent that simply because his parents know he is in therapy does not entitle his parents to know the details of what is being discussed in therapy. In treating older adolescents who may be in college and away from their parents, the psychiatrist does not have as much power in negotiating conditions of treatment. My practice has been to tell such patients that I want their parents to know about their treatment, particularly since at some stage I may want to involve the parents in treatment. I have usually given such patients sufficient time, however, to get used to the idea of their parents' knowing about treatment and have left it up to the patient to inform them.

5

The Psychiatrist's Liability for Negligent Diagnosis

While negligence in the diagnostic process is a common cause of action in most medical specialties, negligent diagnosis in psychiatric practice is rarely alleged or proved. The sparcity of litigation in this area is understandable. There has always been disagreement as to diagnosis in psychiatry. In a field where classifications of diseases as well as definitions of what is and what is not a disease are in a state of constant flux, standards of due care in arriving at a diagnosis are not easily determined. In the absence of such standards it is obviously difficult for a plaintiff to argue that a particular illness was incorrectly diagnosed.

As noted previously, gross negligence on the part of a doctor during the course of commitment proceedings has at times been actionable under the doctrine of negligent diagnosis. Most of the negligent diagnosis actions that have arisen thus far, however, involve suicide or harm to third parties. It is likely that as psychiatric practice becomes more similar to other aspects of medical practice, diagnostic processes will become more scientific and psychiatrists will begin to incur the same risk of liability as other doctors. For this reason some material on negligent diagnosis will be included which covers areas where there thus far have not been any suits, but where litigation might be expected to increase.

If the Psychiatrist Makes an Incorrect Diagnosis and the Patient Is Harmed as a Result, Is the Psychiatrist Automatically Liable?

The psychiatrist is not liable if he used the usual and customary inquiries, examinations, and tests. Suits against psychiatrists in this area would be handled just like suits against any other doctor. A psychiatrist who practices up to current standards including the use of proper laboratory tests and referrals to consultants will not be held liable even if he makes the wrong diagnosis and the patient is thereby harmed. It is worth repeating once again that the general thrust of malpractice law is not to punish the doctor for untoward outcomes, but only for negligence.

Is the Psychiatrist Liable for Failing to Diagnose an Organic Condition?

While I am aware through personal communication of some lawsuits in this area, there are surprisingly no recorded cases in which the psychiatrist has been sued for misdiagnosing an organic condition as a functional illness. (The so-called "functional illnesses" in psychiatry may also have organic determinants. By "organic condition" I mean disease caused by currently measurable anatomical and physiological changes.) Psychiatrists are somewhat more likely to be sued for failing to diagnose a physical illness of a hospitalized patient which may be unrelated to the patient's psychiatric symptoms. The reasons for the paucity of suits involving misdiagnosis of presenting symptoms are not clear. Conceivably, psychiatrists, who are often sensitive about accusations that they are not "real doctors," are extremely careful in diagnosing organicity. Certainly many psychiatrists tend to be extremely cautious and are prone to overdiagnosis of organic conditions. Yet it is unlikely that this is a sufficient explanation of why there has been so little litigation in this area. It is also likely that plaintiffs and their attorneys have simply not appreciated that psychiatrists, like other doctors, are obligated to try to diagnose whatever organic dysfunction may be causing the patient's emotional difficulties.

In theory, psychiatrists should be liable in this area. Certainly psychiatrists who diagnose a patient's symptoms of anxiety or depression as a neurosis and treat it with some form of psychotherapy without thoroughly exploring the patient's physical condition are not practicing up to acceptable standards. Psychiatrists have a clear responsibility to search out organic causes of psychic dysfunction either through their own examinations and work-ups or by referral to competent specialists. As we learn more and more about the manner in which the physical dysfunction produces psychological dysfunction, the psychiatrist assumes an increasing medical obligation to ascertain that the patient's physical condition is thoroughly evaluated.

Is the Psychiatrist Liable for Failing to Diagnose Treatable Side Effects or Complications of Psychiatric Treatment?

The answer here is clearly yes. Side effects or complications are most likely to appear when biological treatments, primarily electroconvulsive therapy (ECT) or psychotropic medications, are utilized. Psychiatrists have been successfully sued for failing to take the diagnostic steps to diagnose a fracture of the spine caused by ECT. [1] Psychotropic medications can cause a wide variety of potentially serious dysfunctions which if diagnosed can be remedied by discontinuing the drug, diminishing the dose, or adding some other treatment. The psychiatrist is in theory liable for failing to diagnose and deal with side effects such as worsening of glaucoma, cardiac dysfunction, incapacitating extrapyramidal symptoms, or severe hypertension which might be related to the administration of various psychotropic drugs. There are no cases reported in these areas as yet, but it is unlikely that this situation will remain static. Conceivably, suits in this area have been raised and settled out of court. As in the case of misdiagnosis of organicity this seems to be an area of malpractice law which will expand as lawyers and plaintiffs gain a greater understanding of the medical responsibilities of psychiatrists.

Under What Circumstances Might Overdiagnosis Lead to a Malpractice Suit?

In the practice of nonpsychiatric medicine a physician who diagnoses a condition that does not exist and treats it in a manner that harms the patient is liable. There have been no similar suits in psychiatry primarily because of the difficulty of defining standards of diagnosis in psychiatric practice. It would be imprudent, however, to assume that plaintiffs and their attorneys will totally ignore this area in the future. Sociologists have repeatedly documented that psychiatrists tend to overdiagnose mental illness.[2] If as the result of such overdiagnosis the patient is subjected to lengthy and expensive treatments which do not help him or is given treatments which actually harm him, there would seem to be a cause of action.

The issue of psychological harm as a result of overdiagnosis has been raised in at least one case.[3] A patient alleged that a psychiatrist and a psychologist had negligently labeled him "paranoid schizophrenic" and caused him humiliation and distress. The court found that the diagnosis had been arrived at with due care and that the term had not been negligently applied. It would have been interesting to know what course the court would have taken if the evidence for the use of due care in

---

[1] L. W. Krouner, "Shock Therapy and Psychiatric Malpractice," *Forensic Sciences* 2, no. 397 (1973): 404; Eisele v. Malone, 2 A.D.2d 550, 157 N.Y.S.2d 155 (1956).
[2] T. J. Scheff, *Being Mentally Ill* (Chicago: Aldine, 1966); S. J. Brakel and R. S. Rock, *The Mentally Disabled and the Law* (Chicago: University of Chicago Press, 1971).
[3] Hendry v. U.S., 418 F.2d 774 (2d Cir. 1969).

arriving at the diagnosis had not been substantial. In this regard it is somewhat frightening to think of the malpractice implications of the Rosenhan article "On Being Sane in Insane Places."[4] This article reported how a group of bogus patients who behaved normally in every way except for describing a single hallucination were all diagnosed as schizophrenic and were treated. Presumably if these had been real patients who were not schizophrenic, and if they had been humiliated and distressed by the labeling process or harmed by subsequent treatment, their doctors would most likely have been liable for negligent diagnosis. As long as the doctor's examination was conducted in a brief and perfunctory manner, the nebulous quality of diagnostic standards in psychiatry might not be a sufficient argument to prevent liability. While it would be difficult to define standards of skill in psychiatric evaluation, it would not be too difficult to define standards of diligence and to determine when a psychiatrist has failed to use due care in being sufficiently diligent.

Are There Situations Where Underdiagnosing a Condition (e.g., Calling a Psychosis a Neurosis or Personality Disorder) Can Lead to Liability?

There are no precedents in this area, but there certainly are a substantial number of psychiatrists who tend to view patients as less sick than most of their colleagues would. As a rule these doctors rely heavily on psychotherapeutic techniques and are reluctant to use drugs and other biological treatments. It is not uncommon for a patient who has received psychotherapy for months or even years without improvement to seek out another doctor and improve rapidly when the new doctor prescribes a biological treatment. It is arguable whether the fault here is negligent diagnosis or negligent treatment, but in any case patients who suffered inordinately because the doctor did not appreciate the severity of their illness might have a cause of legal action. An important consideration here would be the adequacy of the doctor's evaluation. The psychiatric field is sufficiently disorganized, and disagreement between various schools is sufficiently accepted, that unsuccessful outcomes with patients who do not obviously fit into categories are likely to be viewed as nonactionable mistakes in judgment. If the doctor had conducted a negligent evaluation, however, he might be in jeopardy of being sued.

Until recently, many psychiatrists who tended to underdiagnose in terms of the diagnosis placed in the patient's chart felt they were helping their patients by shielding them from the stigma associated with more

[4]D. L. Rosenhan, "On Being Sane in Insane Places," *Science 179* (1973): 250–58.

malignant diagnoses. This has been particularly true of psychiatrists who work with young people in settings such as student health psychiatric clinics. These days the psychiatrist who tries to protect patients in this way may harm the patient and himself. With professional standard review organizations, peer review, and insurance companies demanding that doctors justify their claims, there is a possibility that the patient or the doctor will not be compensated for treatments which third-party payers assume are excessive for the official diagnosis. There is an additional risk that a malpractice suit could be brought alleging that the treatment which was used carried too many risks to be justified in a situation where a relatively benign diagnosis was reported. A psychiatrist would have difficulty justifying the use of large amounts of neuroleptics which produced complications such as tardive dyskinesia with a patient diagnosed as having a neurosis or personality disorder.

Is the Psychiatrist Liable for Failure to Diagnose and Predict Suicide?

In some instances a psychiatrist certainly is liable, but the standards of care in this area are so vague, and court decisions so unpredictable, that it is difficult to offer the practitioner any absolute guidance as to how to avoid liability. In this area of malpractice there is usually clear evidence of damages. The patient is likely to be killed or physically harmed by the suicide attempt. All the plaintiff need prove is that negligence occurred and that it caused the injury. Psychiatrists and mental hospitals have been successfully sued for failing to predict suicide or failing to take proper restraints to prevent suicide once that prediction was made.[5] Suits are brought by plaintiffs who were unsuccessful in committing suicide but managed to injure themselves in the process, or by the relatives of patients who were successful. The issue of failure to take proper precautions might also be considered under the heading of negligent treatment, but for the sake of convenience all malpractice litigation regarding suicide will be discussed in this chapter.

Irwin Perr, an attorney and psychiatrist, notes that when the psychiatrist is held liable for his patient's suicide, the court in effect is asking the psychiatrist to be responsible for someone else's behavior.[6] Except for cases of harm to third parties it is hard to find parallels for this kind of legal reasoning in other aspects of malpractice law. In all other situations

---

[5]I. N. Perr, "Liability of Hospital and Psychiatrist in Suicide," *American Journal of Psychiatry* 122 (1965): 431–638; L. R. Tancredi, J. Lieb, and A. B. Slaby, *Legal Issues in Psychiatric Care* (Hagerstown, Md.: Harper and Row, 1975); I. N. Perr, "Legal Aspects of Suicide," *Legal Aspects of Medical Practice* 6, no. 1 (1978): 49–55.
[6]Perr, "Legal Aspects of Suicide," pp. 49, 53.

the physician is held accountable only for his own or his employees' negligent acts or omissions. A patient hospitalized for treatment of diabetes who is successfully treated may be discharged from the hospital and within a few days become seriously ill by failing to follow the doctor's instructions. No court would impose liability on the physician for such a patient's behavior. The patient would be blamed for not following instructions. A mental patient, however, who has responded well to treatment within the hospital, who is discharged, and who subsequently kills himself is viewed in a different light. Here the patient's relatives may have a cause of action. The blame is shifted to the doctor, and the patient's potential responsibility for his own actions is not fully considered.

The psychiatrist's job is further complicated by legal rulings which require him to treat highly disturbed patients in the least restrictive setting.[7] There is increasing statutory pressure on psychiatrists to release suicidal patients from restrictive settings such as the hospital as soon as possible. Thus, the psychiatrist justifiably feels trapped by the current status of the law with regard to suicide. He has less power than ever to control the actions of a suicidal patient, yet, he still may be liable for what that patient does. The situation is made even worse by our lack of knowledge as to when to use hospitalization and other restraints to prevent suicide. There are few solid criteria by which psychiatrists can diagnose and predict suicidal potential. The best we can do is make rough statements as to the probability of suicide. We may be able to say that a given patient is much more likely to commit suicide than the average citizen, but still the probability of that patient's actually killing himself is quite low. The courts, of course, are unable to determine precisely what degree of probability the psychiatrist has failed to diagnose before he is liable for failing to take action to restrain a suicidal patient. They speak primarily of the psychiatrist's obligation to restrain patients whose suicide is "foreseeable." The vagaries of the term "foreseeable" contribute to the unpredictability of outcome of suicide liability cases.

If the Psychiatrist Is Treating an Outpatient and That Patient Kills Himself, Is the Psychiatrist Liable for Misdiagnosis?

There is certainly a possibility that the psychiatrist in this situation can be sued and, given the vagaries of the law and the unpredictability

---

[7]R. Sadoff, "New Malpractice Concerns for the Psychiatrist," *Legal Aspects of Medical Practice 6*, no. 3 (1978): 31–38.

of juries, the suit might be successful. As a rule, however, the psychiatrist would not be liable unless the indications for suicide had been very powerful, had been communicated to the psychiatrist, and he had failed to take them seriously in making a diagnosis and a treatment disposition. Malpractice suits regarding suicide of outpatients who have not recently been discharged from the hospital are relatively rare. The psychiatrist's liability becomes much greater as he begins to deal with inpatients who commit suicide either in the hospital, shortly after discharge, during leaves of absence, or during unauthorized departures.[8]

If the Psychiatrist Discharges from the Hospital a Patient Whom He Has Been Treating and the Patient Commits Suicide, Is the Psychiatrist at Risk of Liability?

In theory, if the psychiatrist made a careful judgment that the patient had sufficiently improved so as to warrant discharge, the psychiatrist should not be liable. The courts, however, are unpredictable. If the patient was discharged at a time when he had demonstrated signs and symptoms easily observable by the doctor and staff that he was still suicidal, there is a greater chance of a successful lawsuit. A patient who says he is going to kill himself, who has the means of doing so, and who has vegetative signs of depression should obviously not be discharged.

More commonly, the physician is confronted with the patient who seems to be doing well but who, facing the anxiety of leaving the hospital, may hint of suicidal rumination or even make a mild threat. The doctor may feel the patient will be much better off if discharged, but fears a suit if he guesses wrong. Here it is extremely useful for the psychiatrist to write a discharge note in which he states that he has assessed the risks of suicide, has weighed them against the potential advantages of discharge, and has concluded that the benefits are great enough and the risks small enough so that the discharge is clearly warranted. It is even more helpful if a colleague examines the patient and substantiates this opinion. As a general rule any notation in the chart which indicates that the psychiatrist has thought out the risks and benefits of an action taken with regard to the patient diminishes the probability of a lawsuit. If the psychiatrist then turns out to be wrong, he has made a mistake in judgment but has not been negligent. Similar considerations apply to leaves of absence. A well-thought-out risk–benefit note plus timely use of consultation will give as much protection against suits as is possible in this area.

[8]Perr, "Legal Aspects of Suicide," p. 52.

Is the Hospital Liable for the Suicide of the Patient Who Escapes from the Hospital or Who Kills Himself on the Ward?

Where the hospital has been negligent in observing a patient and utilizing reasonable precautions to prevent suicide on the ward or escape, the hospital has been found liable.[9] There, of course, has been considerable controversy as to what constitutes reasonable precaution. In recent years many eminent psychiatrists have advocated limiting the amount of restraint and observation on a psychiatric ward because it is believed that overzealous surveillance impairs successful treatment.[10] The "open door" policy in some psychiatric units is considered a valuable treatment. The therapeutic value of the "open door" policy can be used as an argument to explain the limited surveillance which may have played a part in a hospital suicide or an escape followed by suicide, but it does not provide an absolute shield against liability. Another difficult issue in determining the extent of precautions which must be utilized is the passage of time. A number of people attempt to kill themselves as their condition is improving. If precautions are removed too quickly, the patient may kill himself and the hospital may be liable. Fishalow has noted that the following factors are important for hospitals to consider with regard to the care of suicidal patients:

1. No precise level of patient behavior requires a corresponding level of vigilance. The passage of time dilutes the significance of prior attempts; moreover, there is a somewhat questionable distinction between threats and actual attempts.
2. Watchfulness may be relaxed if the patient's condition improves— but not merely for the sake of expediency.
3. The hospital must maintain its facilities and equipment so that hazards are not created.
4. Staffing ratios if insufficient are from time to time determinative of negligence.
5. Courts will find negligence where it can be proved that the hospital violated its own precautionary rule.
6. If a mistake is found to be an honest error of judgment within a physician's discretion, liability will not usually be assigned.[11]

[9]Mounds Park Hospital v. Von Eye, 245 F.2d 758 (8th Cir. 1957); Benjamin v. Havens, Inc., 60 Wash. 2d 196, 373 P.2d 109 (1962).

[10]Group for the Advancement of Psychiatry, "Toward Therapeutic Care," Report no. 51A (New York: GAP, 1970).

[11]S. G. Fishalow, "The Tort Liability of the Psychiatrist," *Bulletin of the American Academy of Psychiatry and the Law 3*, no. 4 (1975): 205.

Once the Psychiatrist Carefully and on the Basis of Reasonable Evidence Initiates Hospitalization Procedures for the Suicidal Patient, What Are Some Possible Risks of Negligent Malpractice Still to Be Considered?

When a patient is hospitalized for suicidal tendencies, the hospital is obligated to use reasonable efforts to protect that patient from self-harm. Failure on the part of the hospital staff to use sufficient precautions to keep the patient from harming himself frequently results in actions against the hospital. Sometimes a psychiatrist is also named in the suit. The psychiatrist has a clear obligation to inform the hospital staff when he believes there is an imminent risk of the patient's being suicidal. He is obligated to note his judgment and write appropriate orders for the hospital staff to take precautions. The hospital is not responsible for a suicidal act of the patient if its staff did not know that risk.[12] The physician who evaluated the patient has the prime responsibility to inform the staff of the patient's needs.

Are There Other Possible Instances in Which the Psychiatrist Could Be Liable for a Patient's Suicide?

There are at least three other hypothetical scenarios which could result in a lawsuit following a patient's suicide:

1. The doctor might be found liable for allowing the patient access to an unreasonable amount of medication. Certain psychotropic drugs such as tricyclics and monamine oxidase inhibitors (MAOIs) are used to treat the depression of suicidal patients and glutethimide or barbiturates may be used to treat insomnia associated with depression. A relatively small overdose of any of these drugs can be fatal. Physicians are usually wise to restrict the amount of drugs available to suicidal patients. Conceivably, a failure to do so could result in liability.
2. It has been hypothesized that a doctor can so upset a patient by violating confidentiality as to precipitate suicide. (This is an unlikely scenario.)
3. Some suicides may be precipitated by actions of the psychiatrist that are intentional torts, such as battery. Sexual seduction of the patient may lead to deterioration of the patient's emotional state and eventual suicide. It is likely that such situations have actually

[12]Perr, "Legal Aspects of Suicide," p. 52.

developed, but have never been publicized and have never led to documented litigation.

What Effect Does the Threat of Liability for a Patient's Suicide Have on Psychiatric Practice?

There are few aspects of psychiatric practice as difficult as dealing with a suicidal patient. Even with the best possible treatment suicide is not always preventable. The successful suicide of a patient is a devastating experience for the psychiatrist, who is likely to feel a sense of loss, helplessness, anger, and guilt, even though his treatment of the patient was faultless. Any doctor who has ever lost a patient through suicide knows that such an event remains an indelible part of his consciousness. The experiencing may be devastating enough to exert a continuing influence on the psychiatrist's subsequent practice, and sometimes on his personal life. Adding a malpractice suit to the aversive consequences of the patient's suicide can be an especially cruel punishment of the doctor. Yet psychiatrists must live with the constant fear that if a patient kills himself they may face a lawsuit in addition to all the emotional trauma associated with the patient's death.

The fear of a patient's suicide has an insidious influence on many aspects of psychiatric practice. In dealing with the suicidal patient most psychiatrists tend to be overly cautious. Patients believed to be suicidal are hospitalized too frequently and kept in the hospital too long. (Usually the patient is a voluntary participant in unnecessary hospitalization and is merely following the advice of his doctor.) While the hospitalized patient is less likely to commit suicide than the outpatient, there are certain risks incurred by prolonged hospitalization. Patients who are hospitalized too long begin to overestimate the seriousness of their problems. Many learn new illness behaviors in the hospitals, and some become more depressed as a result of prolonged hospitalizations and therefore more suicidal. Hospitalized patients also lose power. Family and friends label them as sick and nonresponsible. Hospitalization may make it more difficult for both patient and doctor to discover how the family is adversely influencing the patient, and it certainly limits the patient's capacity to change the family system constructively.[13]

Another serious problem arises with dependent patients who become convinced that life in the hospital is better than life outside the hospital. These patients soon learn that talk of suicide or self-injury guarantees continued hospitalization. Every psychiatric hospital unit

[13]S. L. Halleck, *The Treatment of Emotional Disorders* (New York: Aronson, 1978).

deals with scores of such patients annually. Their characterological problems are undoubtedly aggravated by their use of the threat of suicide to manipulate the hospital system. Even worse, patients who begin to use suicidal threats and gestures for manipulative purposes may generalize these behaviors to gain control of many types of social situations. They are at high risk of getting in a position where they feel that they must act on their threats. They are also at risk of misjudging the harmfulness of a suicide gesture and killing themselves accidentally. In the absence of data it is difficult to know the extent to which hospitalization saves lives. The clinical experience of most psychiatrists suggests that cautious use of brief hospitalization with acutely disturbed patients is helpful. But there is good reason to doubt that prolonged hospitalization is helpful.

Overconcern about suicide even influences the process of outpatient psychotherapy. The doctor, of course, should communicate to the patient that he cares for him, that he thoroughly disapproves of suicidal behavior, and that he will do whatever he can to prevent the patient's suicide. But this is all he can usefully offer. Too much preoccupation with the issue of suicide prevents the therapist from being as professional as he should be. The psychiatrist preoccupied with the issue of the patient's suicide tends to infantilize the patient. He focuses his attention on protecting the patient rather than helping the patient change. A great deal of psychotherapy in this country degenerates into a dialogue over the extent to which the psychiatrist will intervene to prevent suicide. Usually this is a wasteful dialogue which impedes the process of psychotherapy.

It can, of course, be argued that psychiatrists would be just as preoccupied with the subject of their patients' suicides without the threat of malpractice liability. There is no way of knowing if this is true or false. It would seem, however, that the additive, aversive effects of a malpractice suit are a significant factor in the doctor's overcautiousness.

I am firmly convinced that our legislative bodies would help patients, would save our society millions of dollars, and would improve the quality of practice of psychiatry, if they were to pass laws granting the psychiatrist some immunity from liability for a patient's suicide. Total immunity might be unrealistic since the psychiatrist can get into situations where his duty to protect the patient may be much greater than that of the average person. I doubt that statutory limitations of liability for the patient's suicide will lead to psychiatrists' treating self-destructive patients in a cavalier manner. Psychiatrists will try hard enough to prevent suicide without the fear of malpractice. Diminishing the malpractice threat might turn out to be a significant enough balancing factor to allow the psychiatrist to approach the suicidal patient in a caring, but more rational manner.

What Are the Psychiatrist's Risks of Malpractice When His Patient Injures a Third Party?

The psychiatrist's responsibilities in dealing with a patient who hurts others are similar to those involved in dealing with a patient who hurts himself. If anything, the courts have put even greater liability on psychiatrists and psychiatric hospitals whose patients harm others.[14] Our ability accurately to predict violence toward others is poor, and this reality is well known to scientists and many lawyers. It would, therefore, be difficult to prove that a psychiatrist who simply failed to predict violence and was wrong was negligent. It is only when a psychiatrist has made a prediction of dangerousness and fails to take proper precautions that he risks liability. Most of the cases in this area are directed against hospitals and involve escapes, early discharges, or leaves of absence which result in the patient's harming a third party.[15] As is the case with the issue of suicide, the psychiatrist is again in a position where he has little power to deal with the patient who may commit an antisocial act, but he nevertheless ends up being responsible for the consequences of that patient's actions.

Does a Psychiatrist Have a Legal Obligation to Warn Potential Victims of a Patient's Dangerous Tendencies?

The psychiatrist may not only be liable for failing to impose sufficient restraints on patients who later harm third parties, but may also be liable for failing to inform the injured party as to the probability of an impending assault. Most of the suits involving harm to a third party involve situations in which a patient was already hospitalized and was either unwisely provided with freedom or with the opportunity to escape. Until recently, those few suits based on failure to warn a victim involved hospitalized patients who were released or escaped to situations where it might have benefited others to know of the patient's violent tendencies. Psychiatrists are, as a rule, reluctant to be put into the role of warners or informants since such acts usually require that the patient's confidence be violated. Yet psychiatrists have long had ample ethical support for informing others of the potential dangerousness of their patients. The American Medical Association has formally stated that it is neither a breach of trust nor a violation of professional ethics to

---

[14]Fishalow, "Tort Liability," p. 205.
[15]Weihs v. State, 267 A.D. 233, 45 N.Y.S.2d 542 (1943); St. George v. State, 283 A.D. 245, 127 N.Y.S.2d 147 (1954).

reveal confidential information "where such a breach becomes necessary to protect the welfare of the individuals or the community."[16] This statement supports the psychiatrist's right to inform an intended victim, but it does not obligate the psychiatrist to do so.

The psychiatrist who encounters an outpatient who is diagnosed as potentially violent can try to abort the violent event by initiating commitment of the patient or by warning potential victims. Either action violates confidentiality. A physician who initiates commitment proceedings against a potentially dangerous patient is protected from liability for violating confidentiality in most states.[17] Informing a third person about a patient's violent tendencies, however, provides no statutory immunity and can lead to the patient's suing the doctor for defamation of character. It is unclear to what extent ethical statements such as those of the American Medical Association would protect a psychiatrist in a defamation suit if he overassessed a patient's dangerousness and incorrectly published details of that alleged dangerousness to a third party.

Most of these issues were only of theoretical concern until 1976 when a California court enunciated a ruling which seems to create an obligation for California psychiatrists to inform third parties about their patients' dangerousness. The decision, which has come to be known as the *Tarasoff* ruling, has created a great deal of interest and concern among both psychiatrists and lawyers.[18]

What Are Some of the Facts Involved in the Tarasoff Decision?

A young woman, Tatiana Tarasoff, rejected her suitor, Poddar. Shortly after Poddar had been rejected by Miss Tarasoff, he became emotionally disturbed and entered therapy with a psychologist employed by the University of California at Berkeley Student Health Service. While in therapy, Poddar confided to his therapist his intention to kill Tatiana. The therapist was concerned about this revelation and consulted with his psychiatric colleagues who agreed that Poddar should be committed. The campus police were notified to take Poddar into custody and assist in his commitment. Poddar was apparently able to persuade the police to release him. For some unknown reason, at this point the director of the department of psychiatry at the hospital ordered that no further action be taken and had all correspondence and therapeutic notes related to the case destroyed. No further effort was made to com-

[16]A. Brooks, "Mental Health Law," *Administration in Mental Health*, Fall 1976, p. 95.
[17]R. Slovenko, *Psychiatry and Law* (Boston: Little, Brown, 1973), p. 64.
[18]Tarasoff v. Regents of the University of California, 131 Cal. Rptr. 14 (1976).

mit Poddar. No effort was made to warn Tatiana or anyone close to her of Poddar's threats, and he killed her.

Tatiana's parents brought an action for wrongful death against the psychotherapist, the campus police, and the University of California. The suits against all parties were dismissed in the court of origin. The case was appealed, however, and the California Supreme Court ruled that there was a duty on the part of the therapist to warn Tatiana of the danger, and held that the failure to warn under the circumstances of this case was actionable negligence.[19] The California Supreme Court stated, "When a therapist determines or pursuant to the standards of his profession should determine that his patient presents a serious danger of violence to another he incurs an obligation to use reasonable care to protect the intended victim against such danger." The court reasoned that the therapist stands in some special relationship to either the person whose conduct needs to be controlled or to the foreseeable victim of that conduct. The issue of the therapist's concern as to violating the patient's confidentiality was seriously considered. The court weighed the risks to the patient of violation of confidence against the risk of another person's being injured. It ruled in favor of preventing injury and stated, "the protective privilege ends where the public peril begins."

The *Tarasoff* decision has predictably alarmed psychiatrists and fascinated lawyers. To psychiatrists it represents a new manifestation of potentially oppressive regulation. To lawyers it appears to be a novel legal ruling which opens up a new area of malpractice liability for psychotherapists of all disciplines who have previously been shielded from such risks.

What Are Some of the Concerns Psychiatrists Have Raised about the Tarasoff Decision?

The main arguments which have been invoked against *Tarasoff* are:

1. If psychotherapists have a duty to inform third parties about violent potentialities of patients, certainly patients must be informed at the beginning of therapy that such a duty exists. Providing such information would not only constitute ethical practice, but would be consistent with the doctrine of informed consent. It has been argued that if patients who have problems with violent tendencies are informed at the beginning of therapy that their

---

[19]*Ibid.*

confidentiality can easily be compromised, they will simply not enter therapy. The *Tarasoff* ruling, therefore, may put the public at even greater peril from patients who are potentially violent, but who will go untreated.

2. It is also possible that the patient who has been informed of the therapist's duty to warn will simply not talk about violent tendencies in the therapeutic relationship. This would considerably diminish the value of psychotherapy for these individuals, and if their violent tendencies were untreated would certainly provide the public with little protection.[20]

3. Even if the patient is willing to make full disclosure to a psychiatrist whom he knows may violate such confidences, the potentially violent patient is likely to relate to his psychotherapist with a constant sense of distrust. Without trust in the therapist, the value of therapy would be diminished. The violent patient would be unlikely to improve and would remain a risk to the public.[21]

4. Conceivably, one of the easy ways out of the duty to inform would be simply to try to initiate commitment of any patient who shows hints of violent tendencies. If the patient is hospitalized, danger to third parties is minimized and the responsibility for the patient's disposition may be in someone else's hands. (If the court releases the patient, there is an assumption that the patient has been adjudicated nondangerous and it would then be difficult to blame the psychiatrist for the patient's subsequent violence.) The *Tarasoff* decision could lead to more unnecessary civil commitments. Since in California (and many other states) it is increasingly difficult to retain the potentially violent patient in the hospital for more than a few days, such a patient might soon be released. He would return to a treatment situation where his relationship with the therapist would now be tenuous, or if the patient feels sufficiently betrayed, nonexistent.

5. Therapists could overreact and practice defensively by warning too often. It is a rare patient in any form of therapy who does not express aggressive and even violent tendencies at some time or another. Even relatively normal people undergoing psychoanalysis often express murderous feelings toward their parents, children, or spouse. The worst vision of the critics of *Tarasoff*

---

[20]H. Gurevitz: "Protective Privilege Versus Public Peril," *American Journal of Psychiatry 134*, no. 3 (1977): 289–92.

[21]A. A. Stone, "The Tarasoff Decision: Suing Psychiatrists to Safeguard Society," *Harvard Law Review 90*, no. 2 (1976): 358–78.

is that therapists would be threatened to warn third parties every time they heard such communications.[22]

6. Psychiatrists are naturally concerned that they can be sued for failure to warn and also be sued for defamation of character if they do warn. The guidelines which would cover either kind of suit are unclear. The California Supreme Court asked only for a reasonable degree of skill, knowledge, and care in making decisions to warn, but such a statement does not provide clear guidelines as to what doctors must do to protect themselves from liability.

To all of the above concerns I would add that this is another situation in which psychiatrists have been put in the situation where they have less power and more responsibility. In the days when civil commitment was easily accomplished, the issue of duty to warn was not likely to be too important. The patient could be kept in a protective setting. Now the psychiatrist has much less control over the patient yet he has more liability for the patient's actions.

Finally, it should be noted that the *Tarasoff* ruling declares that the therapist may be liable in instances where he should determine that his patient presents a danger to others. The term "should" here implies that the therapist is capable of making such determinations and can be viewed as being negligent if he fails to perform up to the standards of his profession in this task. Yet there is overwhelming evidence that there are no useful standards for predicting dangerousness.[23] The court seems to be saying that psychiatrists can be held negligent for failing to perform competently in an area in which the profession has little or no expertise. Again, psychiatrists experience such demands as oppressive.

How Is the Tarasoff Decision Liable to Affect Psychiatric Practice?

The *Tarasoff* ruling involved a very unusual case which is likely to have less impact than most psychiatrists fear. First of all, it applies only in the state of California. Second, it involves a situation in which the psychiatrist had made a clear prediction of danger and had done it publicly by informing the police. The best judgment of the psychiatrist involved in this case was that the patient was dangerous. The psychia-

---

[22]L. H. Roth and A. Meisel, "Dangerousness, Confidentiality and the Duty to Warn," *American Journal of Psychiatry 134*, no. 5 (1977): 508–11.

[23]C. J. Frederick, ed. *Dangerous Behavior: A Problem in Law and Mental Health*, DHEW Publication no. 78–563 (Washington, D.C.: DHEW, 1978).

trist in private practice who does not feel that the patient who makes aggressive threats is truly going to carry them out, or who believes that the risks of violence on the part of the patient are minimal, can simply state this in his notes and it would seem that he would be protected from liability. Recall, it is only when the psychiatrist has already predicted dangerousness, or should have predicted it, that there is a duty to warn. The doctor's notes can reflect that no dangerousness was predicted. Given the enormous amount of expert opinion as to the difficulty of predicting dangerousness, the "should have" provision would also seem to pose very little threat to the psychiatrist who simply stated that dangerousness was unlikely. In equivocal cases the written agreement of a colleague would provide even more protection.

The *Tarasoff* decision has not thus far led to similar successful litigation in other states. Even in California, a recent suit attempting to establish that a psychiatrist had a duty to warn family members about a patient's potentiality for suicide was defeated.[24]

While it is much too early to predict the eventual outcome of *Tarasoff* on psychiatric practice, my best guess is that its major effects will be a slight diminution in the quality of care of potentially violent patients (in large part because psychiatrists will be less willing to treat them) and an occasional lawsuit against a psychiatrist for defamation of character. These are not insignificant consequences, but are probably far less drastic than psychiatrists first envisioned.

In the course of studying the *Tarasoff* decision I have had personal experiences which lead me to question its implied rationale that the potential victim is in a substantially better position if warned. About a year after the *Tarasoff* court reaffirmed its decision I received a note from a colleague telling me that a patient had made statements to her that seemed to indicate that he was planning to kill me. My colleague, apparently responding to her perception of the *Tarasoff* ruling, felt that it was her duty to warn me even though there has been no such ruling in my state. I received the information as to the possible threat against my life with some consternation and much confusion. In pondering what I could do about the threat, I realized that there were few possibilities. I could leave town, but I knew that the patient, who was a student, would be in town for several years. I could have bought a gun and kept it at home or in my office, but I found this alternative distasteful and in conflict with my values. I finally did the only thing that seemed to make sense—I called the police. They agreed to drive by my house every now and then, and advised me to change my habits so that I would not be predictably in the same place all the time. They asked my opinion as to

24Bellah v. Greenson, 1 Cir. No. 39770. (Cal. Oct. 5, 1977.)

whether I thought they should talk to the patient and tell him to stay away from me. I thought this was a good idea and they complied. Nothing more came of the matter, but I must admit that I was overly anxious, hyperalert, and much more aggressive than I usually am during the ensuing few months. The emotional trauma I experienced by being warned, while not overwhelming, was in no way worth the very doubtful benefits I accrued by having been warned. I now fear that if we ever do get to the point of warning all people who are threatened, we will probably not save many lives but we will certainly cause a great deal of mental anguish.

Although warnings may be useless, there are ways of providing them without imposing a threat of liability upon doctors. A law could be written which would require the psychiatrist to report serious threats of violence in patients who are unlikely to be civilly committed directly to a magistrate. The court would then have the opportunity to weigh the psychiatrist's report and make a legal decision as to whether the threat was serious enough to warrant violating the patient's confidentiality. It would seem that decisions to warn in this kind of setting would be more rational since they would have the input of legal as well as psychiatric wisdom. Liability would not be an issue since the decision-making power would rest with the magistrate, who could not be sued.

6

The Psychiatrist's Liability for Negligence in the Process of Consent and Treatment

Like all other doctors, according to law the psychiatrist must obtain consent from patients before initiating diagnostic procedures or treatment. Initiating procedures with patients who have not consented to treatment may be actionable under the law of battery. But even if the patient does agree to a particular intervention, the physician can still be sued if he has been negligent in providing sufficient information as to the risks of that procedure. Lawsuits based on the physician's failure to provide adequate information to the patient are usually adjudicated under the theory of negligence. The physician can be liable not only for treating without consent, but also for treating when the patient consents without having received sufficient information.

Once a valid and informed consent has been obtained, the psychiatrist can still be sued for negligent provision of treatment. As is the case with regard to negligent diagnosis, suits involving negligent treatment are rare in psychiatry. It is extremely difficult to determine what is negligent treatment in psychiatry. Standards governing the use of our treatments are nebulous and agreement as to what is the most effective treatment for a given disorder is not overly common. Most psychiatric conditions are treated with a variety of interventions by different practitioners. Even the same intervention can be used quite differently by one practitioner than by another.

Most of the litigation regarding negligent psychiatric treatment involves biological or somatic treatment. As psychiatrists practice more like other doctors, they begin to incur the same malpractice risks as other doctors. It is interesting to note, however, that as electroconvulsive therapy has become more efficient and less risky (and more difficult to provide because of legal restraints), lawsuits involving its use seem to be diminishing. There have been only a few suits regarding negligent use of psychotropic drugs, but there is every reason to anticipate that this situation will change. Given the seemingly infinite variety of behaviors that are justified as therapeutic by one school of psychotherapy or another, there is, as might be expected, a paucity of cases involving negligent psychotherapy. Only a few cases are regularly discussed in the literature, and in all instances they are characterized by extremely deviant practices on the part of the defendant.

It is not uncommon in psychiatric practice for the patient to be terminated from treatment without having achieved cure or substantial improvement. There is some question as to whether some psychiatrists may be risking malpractice suits under the doctrine of abandonment when they make unilateral decisions to terminate treatment. There are no recorded cases in this area, but the issue does warrant consideration.

What Are the Legal Elements Involved in Obtaining Consent to Treatment?

The three major elements of consent are capacity, voluntariness, and information. The term "capacity" is usually equated with the term "competency." As a rule, the patient who consents to a given procedure or treatment is presumed to be competent unless the issue of incompetence is raised. It is also usually assumed that the patient who consents to treatment is doing so on a voluntary basis unless the voluntariness of the consent is questioned. The need for information is based on the doctrine that the physician may not treat a patient until he has explained to the patient the risk and material facts concerning the treatment and its alternatives, including nontreatment, and has secured the patient's consent based on the patient's understanding of that information.

What Are the Major Malpractice Issues Related to Capacity or Competency to Consent?

The issue as to whether a patient is competent or incompetent arises in many legal settings other than those dealing with consent to treatment. Some of the more general issues involving legal competency and the right to refuse treatment will be discussed in other chapters. Here I will focus primarily on the risks of malpractice the psychiatrist incurs in treating patients whose competency to accept or refuse treatment is in doubt. Whenever a patient has a serious mental illness which interferes with his cognitive functioning, his perception, or his capacity to behave in a self-serving manner, the question of his competency to accept or refuse treatment is always at issue. There is a tendency among psychiatrists and other physicians automatically to assume that those patients who go along with our recommendations for treatment are competent and to raise the question of incompetence only when the patient questions our judgment. (Psychiatrists are not too different from other professionals in this regard. I have noted that lawyers rarely worry about the competence of their clients as long as legal advice is followed. It is only when the client questions the attorney's wisdom by refusing to plea bargain or by disagreeing with other aspects of the attorney's strategy that the attorney begins to suspect incompetence.) As a general rule, we have been conditioned to view an affirmative response to the recommendation of a professional as rational and tend to suspect incompetency only when the response is negative. Obviously, there is something overly paternalistic and inconsistent about this approach. Psychiatrists should be concerned with the competency of consenting as well as nonconsenting patients.

In evaluating the competency of the patient's consent or lack of consent, there are four possible situations which should be considered:

1. The patient agrees to treatment and seems to be competent to make that decision.
2. The patient refuses treatment and seems to be competent in making that refusal.
3. The patient agrees to treatment but his competency is in doubt.
4. The patient refuses treatment and his competency is in doubt.[1]

In the first instance there is no problem. There are no risks of a lawsuit when a competent patient consents to treatment as long as the other conditions of voluntariness and adequate provision of information are met. There are important issues for the psychiatrist to consider, however, if a patient presumed to be competent rejects treatment. Often patients who may have fairly severe mental illnesses seem to have a fairly good understanding of their illness and the implications of treatment, and it is usually clear to the psychiatrist that no court would find them incompetent. Sometimes these patients may even be committed to the hospital on an involuntary status. In past years psychiatrists often treated these patients without consent. Usually the patients were involuntarily committed and it was assumed that the patient who could not make a competent decision as to whether or not he needed hos-

[1]L. H. Roth, A. Meisel, and C. W. Lidz, "Tests of Competency to Consent to Treatment," *American Journal of Psychiatry 134*, no. 3, (1977): 279–83.

pitalization could not make a competent decision with regard to treatment. Today this kind of reasoning is not accepted by legislators or by courts.[2] Some statutes specifically prohibit the use of electroconvulsive therapy with competent nonconsenting patients.[3] Some courts have ruled that committed patients who have not been found incompetent cannot be treated with neuroleptic drugs against their will.[4] It has been argued that in states where the statutory standards that govern commitment imply that the patient must be incompetent to be involuntarily hospitalized, or where the statute requires that the patient must be treated, the psychiatrist incurs little risk by treating a nonconsenting committed patient with neuroleptics.[5] But even here caution is essential since the patient has not been formally adjudicated incompetent. The psychiatrist may still be at risk of being sued under a federal statute (section 1983 of the U.S. Code, a civil rights statute) which deals with the violation of civil rights under the color of law. Doctors who treat involuntary patients do act under the color of the law, and the federal statute which governs this issue allows suits for damages against those who, acting under the color of the law, deprive persons of their civil liberties. If the psychiatrist practices in a state where the standards for commitment do not include reference to the patient's incompetency or to the necessity of providing treatment, the psychiatrist is in even greater jeopardy if he treats a nonconsenting patient.

Until quite recently psychiatrists assumed that the consent of a close relative was sufficient to allow for treatment of a committed or noncommitted patient even though the patient was not formally adjudicated incompetent. These days it should be clear that such consent is of little value in justifying involuntary treatment and does not protect the psychiatrist from malpractice. Family members can legally overrule the patient's refusal to accept treatment only when the patient has been adjudicated incompetent and they are appointed as his guardian.[6]

It is not uncommon for patients whose competency is very much in doubt to consent to treatment. They may manifest such consent verbally or may simply say nothing and proceed to cooperate with treatment. (Patients who do not indicate a choice as to whether they do or do not desire treatment are assumed to be incompetent. It is legally safe to treat them when the proper indications are present.) As noted previously, psychiatrists do not often question the competency of patients who consent to treatment. To provide maximum protection to the patient and

[2]A. Brooks, "The Right to Refuse Treatment," *Administration in Mental Health 4*, no. 2 (1977): 90–94.

[3]Vasconcellos Bill, California State Assembly Bill 4481.

[4]L. H. Roth, "Judicial Action Report," *Psychiatric News 14*, no. 9 (1979): 3.

[5]Brooks, "Right to Refuse Treatment," p. 90

[6]B. J. Ennis, nd R. D. Emery, *The Rights of Mental Patients* (New York: Avon Books, 1978).

himself, the doctor should always question any severely disturbed patient's acceptance of treatment. When the doctor suspects that a patient who is accepting treatment is incompetent, there is some value in having the patient's next of kin agree to the treatment plan and sign a written form acknowledging that agreement. Another possibility available in some states is to obtain a court injunction which certifies that the patient's consent in this particular instance is competent. Courts as a rule will not demand a high standard of competence when the patient willingly accepts a treatment that doctors feel is highly indicated. A third and certainly much more complicated procedure is to have the patient declared incompetent, have a guardian appointed, and have the guardian consent to treatment. Ultimately, this is the most consistent and legally sound action the doctor can take.[7] Unfortunately, it requires delays and a commitment of the doctor's time which may interfere with good clinical practice. While there have been no malpractice suits thus far in this area, it would seem desirable that physicians at least obtain the written consent of the patient's next of kin when they have doubts as to the consenting patient's competency to agree to a given treatment.

The most difficult problem the psychiatrist encounters in day-to-day work is in dealing with the patient who refuses a given treatment, but whose competency is very much in doubt. Certainly, if that patient is in an emergency situation where his life is threatened, customary medical treatment can be instituted against the patient's will through emergency commitment proceedings or emergency incompetency proceedings (some states have developed statutes which allow for an emergency declaration of incompetency when the patient's life is threatened). It has been previously noted that in some states a committed patient can be treated against his will, and in most states a committed patient behaving in a manner which endangers the safety of himself or others may be treated against his will. As a general rule, however, the doctor is on much safer grounds if he delays treatment of a nonconsenting patient whose competency is in doubt until the patient is adjudicated incompetent.

While the physician must always be cautious in treating nonconsenting patients, there are also malpractice precedents which suggest that the physician may be obligated to treat nonconsenting patients who need treatment but who are incompetent. In one case the court ruled that failure to treat an incompetent patient mainly because the patient refused treatment was "illogical, unprofessional, and non-consistent with medical standards."[8]

[7] R. H. Turnbull, *The Law and the Mentally Handicapped in North Carolina*, Chapel Hill: Institute of Government, University of North Carolina, (1979).
[8] Whitree v. State, 56 Misc. 2d 693, 290 N.Y.S.2d 486 (1968).

In nonpsychiatric medicine, there is one important case in which a doctor was successfully sued for failing to perform surgery on a patient who was heavily sedated, semiconscious, and refusing treatment. The patient eventually lost all the toes on one foot because of the doctor's failure to operate. She testified at the trial that she had no recollection of ever being asked to consent to treatment. In this case the court ruled that the physician was legally required to consult the patient's next of kin and obtain their approval for surgery.[9] This case dates back to 1959. Conceivably, in today's civil-rights-oriented society the doctor would more likely be held responsible to ascertain that procedures were initiated to declare the patient incompetent and have a guardian appointed who could legally consent to the patient's treatment.

The above considerations suggest that psychiatrists are in an interesting dilemma when confronted with patients who are probably incompetent and who refuse treatment, but whose refusal does not lead to dire physical consequences. Many psychotic individuals these days refuse treatment. Patients diagnosed as having manic-depressive disorders are especially likely to do so. Such patients are not usually committable under current standards which require a finding of dangerousness to self or others. The untreated illnesses of these individuals does not usually lead to physical deterioration, but frequently does lead to psychological and social deterioration. There is no legal justification for treating these patients involuntarily unless they have been adjudicated incompetent. As a rule psychiatrists do not go through the tedious process of initiating incompetency proceedings with this type of patient. Nor are we usually diligent in advising family members of the possibility of using the incompetency procedure as a means of having their disturbed relative treated. In this area we may be courting malpractice suits by being too "civil rights minded" and failing to make full and proper use of laws covering incompetency and the appointment of guardians. The patient and family who lose dignity, community status, and wealth as a result of the patient's erratic behavior during an acute phase of a manic illness could conceivably sue the doctor for not pursuing a declaration of the patient's incompetency or for failing to advise them of guardianship laws which would have allowed them to have sought to have the patient adjudicated incompetent.

What Is Meant by "Voluntariness" of Consent?

It is usually presumed that the person who consents to treatment does so voluntarily. There are situations, however, in which the patient

9Steele v. Woods, 327 S.W.2d 187 (Mo. 1959).

agrees to treatment because he is subjected to some form of constraint or coercion. Institutionalized patients are at special risk of being coerced to accept treatments because of external persuasion or compulsion. The patient may be promised certain rewards if he consents to treatment and certain punishments if he does not. Concern over the voluntariness of the hospitalized mental patient's consent has arisen with regard to experimental projects involving psychosurgery and behavior modification in both correctional and mental health institutions. In a number of instances courts have ruled that patients confined to highly restrictive situations cannot "volunteer" for certain treatments.[10]

Psychiatrists as individual practitioners have thus far not been subject to malpractice suits for coercing treatment. It must be noted, however, that hospital-employed psychiatrists are sometimes "heavy handed" in making promises as to the rewards which will follow acceptance of treatment and threats as to punishments that might follow nonacceptance. This is certainly a borderline area. When we tell a patient that we will release him from the hospital if he consents to receive an injection of prolixin there is a certain element of coercion involved; but we may also be trying to serve the best interests of the patient by responding to the reality that the patient might be unwilling to take short-acting medication and could not stay out of the hospital without the benefit of long-acting medication. Given the nature of psychiatric practice there will always be ill-defined rewards available to the patient who accepts treatment and does well, and subtle aversive consequences to the patient who refuses treatment and does poorly. It would seem that the most reasonable course for psychiatrists to follow is to explain the contingencies involved in refusing or not refusing treatment in as matter-of-fact a manner as possible and without making exorbitant promises or threats. (It might be noted that the courts are as likely to coerce "voluntary treatment" as psychiatrists. I have on several occasions observed judges' telling competent patients that they would be involuntarily committed if they did not "volunteer" to accept outpatient pharmacological or psychotherapeutic interventions.)

What Issues Are Involved in Providing Information to the Patient?

If the physician were functioning only as a businessman and related to patients entirely on a contractual or fee-for-service basis, the patient's competency and voluntariness would be sufficient conditions for con-

[10]B. Barber *et al., Research on Human Subjects: Problems of Social Control in Medical Experimentation* (New York: Russell Sage Foundation, 1973); Kaimowitz for John Doe v. Michigan Department of Mental Health, Civ. no. 73-19453-4 (1973).

sent. But the doctor's responsibility is greater than the businessman's. Because the doctor is so much more knowledgable than the patient regarding medical matters, he owes the patient a special or "fiduciary" duty. The doctor must look out for the patient's welfare. One way of doing this is by providing him with information regarding treatment. In medical practice the patient's consent is not completed unless it is based on his having been provided with information as to the risks and material facts concerning the treatment, including nontreatment. When we say that information is a prerequisite of consent we are formulating a legal principle that is loosely referred to as "the doctrine of informed consent."

When the patient makes a competent and voluntary agreement to undertake a given procedure for treatment there is still a possibility of malpractice if the doctor has not provided sufficient information about the treatment to the patient and the patient is treated and subsequently harmed. Here the doctor's liability is for negligence. Because of the fiduciary nature of the doctor–patient relationship the doctor has an affirmative duty to the patient to disclose relevant material as to the risks of treatment. If these are not disclosed and the patient suffers one of these risks, the doctor's failure to provide such information can be viewed as the proximate cause of the patient's harm. The reasoning here is that the patient may not have agreed to undertake the treatment if he had been fully aware of the risks.

The doctrine of informed consent is primarily designed to protect the patient's right of self-determination. It is assumed that an adult who is competent has the right to determine whether or not to submit to medical treatment. Or in the often-quoted words of Justice Cardoza, "Every human being of adult years and sound mind has a right to determine what shall be done to his body."[11] Some additional reasons often cited for the value of the informed consent doctrine is that greater information allows for better decision-making on the part of the patients and that sharing of information also makes for a more egalitarian doctor–patient relationship in which the patient is more likely to be a participant in his own treatment.[12]

The doctrine of informed consent is very important in psychiatric practice. One of the major decisions that led to a recent renewal of interest in the informed consent doctrine involved psychiatric treatment.[13] A patient received insulin and electroconvulsive therapy for the

---

[11]Schloendorff v. Society of N.Y. Hospital, 211 N.Y. 125, 105 N.E. 92 (N.Y. 1914).
[12]G. J. Annas, *The Rights of Hospital Patients* (New York: Avon Books, 1975), p. 57.
[13]Mitchell v. Robinson, 334 S.W.2d 11 (Mo. 1960); *affd. after retrial*, 360 S.W. 673 (Mo. 1962).

treatment of schizophrenia. The treatment caused the fracture of several vertebrae. Even though the patient had consented to treatment, the court ruled that the patient's consent was insufficient to shield the doctor from liability for the harmful results. The consent was judged invalid in this case because the physician did not inform the patient thoroughly of the possible hazards of the treatment.

What Kind of Information Regarding Treatment Should Be Provided to Psychiatric Patients?

As a general rule a patient should be informed whenever possible as to the major risks, discomforts, and side effects of treatment. In most instances thorough provision of information to the patient is good medical practice as well as good legal practice. A patient on neuroleptic medication, for example, who is warned that he may experience symptoms associated with extrapyramidal and autonomic nervous system changes will be better able to cooperate with his doctor in treating these side effects. Many doctors are extremely diligent in informing patients about risks and side effects simply because providing such information facilitates treatment.

If the patient is to make a rational decision as to whether or not he wants to undertake the risks of a given therapy, he should also know the benefits of that treatment. A discussion of risk–benefit ratios of treatment would seem to be an integral part of good medical care. Knowledge of potential benefits increases the patient's hope and optimisim. Knowledge as to the limits of potential benefits is also helpful. The patient who knows that a given treatment will ameliorate rather than cure is unlikely to become disturbed when he discovers that treatment dose not totally rid him of discomfort.

The patient should also be informed to the best of the physician's knowledge as to what might happen if no treatment at all is provided. Such information is merely a statement of the patient's prognosis. When there is more than one treatment for a given condition, it is also prudent for the physician to point out the existence of alternative treatments. This is especially useful in dealing with relatively intact patients. A phobic patient, for example, who might be treated with behavior modification, tricyclics, or long-term psychotherapy, should know that all of these interventions are available and should know why the physician prefers to use a particular treatment or combination of treatments. The discussion of alternative treatments with the patient gives the physician an opportunity to provide the patient with rational reasons why one treatment may be better than another.

In a later section I will note instances in which too much disclosure
of information may be bad for patients. When the doctor restricts information to help the patient, his good medical practice may leave him
open to a lawsuit. But as a general rule the doctrine of informed consent
is quite compatible with good medical practice.

Is the Method of Disclosure of Information Important?

The manner in which information is presented to the patient is as
important as the substance or the content of disclosure.[14] The physician
is obligated to present information in a way which maximizes the probability that it will be received and understood. It is important that the
physician try to avoid jargon and provide information which the patient
is capable of comprehending. Explanation of risk must be tailored carefully to meet the intellectual capacities of the patient. It is also important
that the explanation be tailored to the patient's language abilities. If a
patient does not have a good understanding of English, it is important
that information be given in his native language, and where necessary a
translator should be used. If information is presented to the patient in
written form, it should be expressed as simply and clearly as possible
and be in large print. Finally, once the information has been presented
the doctor should offer to answer any questions the patient might have.

How Much Understanding of the Communicated Information Must the Patient Have?

The courts have urged doctors to ascertain that information is not
only communicated to the patient, but also understood by the patient.
Yet it is unclear how the physician might go about assessing a patient's
level of understanding, and it is also uncertain if the physician is obligated to make such an evaluation. There are certainly no standards
developed either by the medical profession or by the courts which
evaluate the patient's level of understanding. There have been suits
brought as battery charges against surgeons who used terminology the
patient misunderstood and who then proceeded to perform surgical
procedures far more drastic than the patient anticipated.[15] In these
cases, however, there is more of a quality of the patient's being misled

[14]Cobbs v. Grant, 8 Cal. 3d 229, 502 P.2d 1 (1972).
[15]Gray v. Grunnell, 423 Pa. 144, 223 A.2d 663 (1966).

than a failure to be concerned with the degree of the patient's under-standing.

The issue of how much understanding the patient needs to provide an informed consent remains murky. So far the courts have focused on the transmission of information rather than on its reception and assimi-lation. If the information transmitted is such that a reasonable person would have received and assimilated it, the consent decision is valid.[16] Problems could certainly arise if the patient were unable to receive and assimilate information as a reasonable person would. Theoretically this could happen if the patient's sensorium were clouded by illness or medication, if the patient had a hearing or language problem, or if the patient had a mental illness. The issue of mental illness brings us right back to the question of competency. A mentally ill patient who cannot receive and assimilate information relevant to treatment is not compe-tent to make a reasonable decision regarding treatment. Faulty com-prehension of information regarding treatment can lead to an incompe-tent acceptance or an incompetent refusal of treatment.

If the doctor suspects that the patient who is agreeing to receive treatment does not really understand the risks and benefits of treatment it would be wise either to have the patient adjudicated incompetent or inform the patient's relatives fully as to the consequences of treatment and to obtain their consent to treatment. If the patient is refusing treat-ment, it would be unlikely that treatment would be given unless the patient were civilly committed and/or declared incompetent. Treatment of a committed patient presumed to be incompetent or of a patient adjudicated incompetent should not be instituted without the informed consent of the next of kin. If the patient is committed and presumed to be incompetent, or is actually adjudicated incompetent, the patient's nearest relative or guardian must be the person who consents to treat-ment. It is then critical that the relative or guardian receive all the infor-mation that would have been given to a competent patient.

What Are Some Limiting Factors in Providing Information to Psychiatric Patients?

In actual practice psychiatrists find it difficult to be comprehensive in providing information, particularly to psychotic patients. The most common treatment used with psychotic patients is neuroleptic medica-tion. There are few psychiatrists who at the time of giving neuroleptics

---

[16]U.S. Department of Health, Education and Welfare, "Protection of Human Subjects: Proposed Policy," *Federal Register 39* (August 1974): 30647-30557.

to a psychotic patient recite all the possible adverse side effects these drugs can produce. Many psychotic patients would be incapable of understanding this information if it were provided. Others would be frightened and further upset by hearing about complications and side effects. As will be noted later, the psychiatrist has some privilege not to disclose information to certain emotionally disturbed patients. This makes good sense in many situations. There is some question, however, if we are under an obligation to discuss the risks and benefits of neuroleptic treatment with the severely disturbed patient's next of kin. Psychiatrists may be leaving themselves open for lawsuits in this area. There is a critical need to develop practices for dealing with informed consent of psychotic patients that are good for the patient and protect the psychiatrist.

One method of practice I have found to be useful is to provide the psychotic patient with only that information as to risks and side effects which I believe he can assimilate and which he should know about if he is to be an effective participant in the treatment process. Most psychotic patients need to know about immediate side effects related to the autonomic and extrapyramidal nervous system, and many can understand these warnings. I try routinely to warn patients started on neuroleptics about symptoms such as stuffy nose, dry mouth, blurred vision, or constipation, and I place particular emphasis on warning them about postural hypotension, akinesia, dystonia, and akathisia. The longer range side effects such as sexual dysfunction, depression, blood dyscrasia, hepatitis, seizures, and particularly tardive dyskinesias, are not discussed with the patient until he is much better, has developed a therapeutic alliance with me, and can make a more rational risk–benefit decision. Once the patient is out of the hospital, he must also of course be warned as to how his medication is influenced by other intercurrent illnesses and by use of other kinds of medications.

I try to inform the acutely psychotic patient's relatives about all the side effects of neuroleptic treatment including tardive dyskinesias. It is helpful to have a printed form which lists all side effects and risks of neuroleptic medication in a clear and succinct manner. It can be read by the patient's relatives when the patient is too disturbed to understand it and then be read by the patient when his psychosis is under control.

What Standards Are the Courts Currently Using in Malpractice Suits Involving Informed Consent?

The current trend is for the courts to demand that the doctor provide as much information as possible. The limiting factors in provision of information, however, are not clearly defined. In one major decision the court noted, "There is no duty to discuss the relatively minor risks inherent in common procedures when it is common knowledge that such risks are of very low incidence."[17] The drawing of blood was mentioned by the court as a procedure in which the risks are common knowledge and of low incidence. The courts have insisted that there is no demand for doctors to discuss minor risks. Legal definitions of minor risks, however, are disturbingly capricious. In one case in which a child contracted polio from an oral vaccine, the court ruled that a risk incidence of one in almost six million should have been revealed.[18]

The theories used by courts to define standards of disclosure are shifting toward greater disclosure. It is no longer safe to assume that the physician should disclose only what other physicians practicing in the same community might disclose. When current standards focus on physician's skills, they require that the amount of information revealed be that which a reasonably skilled physician would offer, and not what other physicians in the community do offer. There is an even more recent trend for the courts to focus not on the skill and diligence of the doctor but on the needs of the patient. Courts have ruled that the duty to disclose should not be defined by the practice of other doctors, but should be a function of the patient's right of self-decision. In other words, whatever information a reasonable patient would need to know to make an informed decision must be provided.[19]

Under What Circumstances May a Doctor Withhold Relevant Information from a Competent Adult Patient?

When a patient is fully competent, the psychiatrist's therapeutic privilege not to disclose information regarding risks of therapy is limited. If the disclosure of all facts, diagnoses, and alternatives or possibilities that might occur to the doctor could so alarm the patient that it would constitute bad medical practice, such disclosure would be unwarranted. Conceivably, too much disclosure might so upset the patient as to increase the risk of utilizing the treatment. While the doctor may restrict disclosure in order to help the patient, it is not allowable to withhold information regarding risks out of the simple motivation of getting the patient to accept treatment. This area, however, is murky.

---

[17]Cobbs v. Grant, 8 Cal. 3d 229, 502 P.2d 1 (1972).
[18]Reyes v. Wyeth Laboratories, 498 F.2d 1264 (5th Cir. 1974).
[19]Cobbs v. Grant, 8 Cal. 3d 229, 502 P.2d 1 (1972); Canterbury v. Spence, 464 F.2d 772 (D.C. Cir. 1972).

The California Supreme Court has ruled that information can be limited when its provision would so seriously upset the patient that the patient would not have been able dispassionately to weigh the risks of refusing to undergo the recommended treatment.[20]

There seem to be no malpractice risks for the doctor in providing maximum disclosure. No doctor has ever been sued for providing too much accurate information.

For the sake of completeness it should be noted that a competent patient has the right to ask not to be told about the risks of treatment. The courts have ruled that "A medical doctor need not make disclosure of risks when the patient requests that he not be so informed."[21] In this situation it is important that the doctor be relatively certain of the patient's competence. It is also wise to have the patient sign a statement which indicates the patient's willingness to waive the right to be fully informed.

How Have Suits Involving Informed Consent Influenced Psychiatric Practice in the Past, and How Are They Likely to Influence Psychiatric Practice in the Future?

The earlier cases involving informed consent in psychiatry were related to the use of electroconvulsive treatment (ECT). In some cases where little or no information was provided to the patient or to relatives the plaintiff's suits were successful. In other cases involving the use of ECT the main issue was whether a spouse or parent could provide informed consent for the patient even though the patient had not been adjudicated incompetent. In all cases prior to 1964 the courts ruled that the "good faith" consent of a relative (presumably based on adequate provision of information) was sufficient to shield the physician from liability.[22] There are no recent cases involving this type of situation, but in view of the new civil rights litigation in this decade and the emergence of the doctrine of a right to refuse treatment, it is unlikely that similar rulings would still be possible. In general, physicians have learned to be extremely careful in obtaining informed consent to the use of electroconvulsive treatment and indeed are often required by law to be especially cautious. In many states the procedure can never be legally

---

[20]Annas, *Rights of Hospital Patients*, p. 67.
[21]Cobbs v. Grant, 8 Cal. 3d 229, 502 P.2d 1 (1972).
[22]S. E. Fishalow, "The Tort Liability of the Psychiatrist," *Bulletin of the American Academy of Psychiatry and the Law 3*, no. 4, (1975): 196.

used with a nonconsenting patient unless the patient is declared incompetent.[23]

Because of new statutory regulations and new rulings regarding the right to refuse treatment, it seems unlikely that we will see further informed consent suits related to ECT. When ECT is used at all these days the psychiatrist tends to be unusually prudent in disclosing risks. Another reason for an anticipated decrease of such suits is that even in an informed consent suit there has to be some harm to the patient and modern-day ECT has become a treatment which rarely results in injury.

In spite of the safety of modern-day ECT it should hardly be necessary to remind psychiatrists that telling patients that shock treatments are perfectly safe and incur no risk whatsoever is foolhardy. Such statements not only fail to meet the doctrine of informed consent, but can also be viewed as implied promises or warranties which might expose the physician to liability under the law of contracts.

There is very little recorded case law involving suits related to failure to inform patients as to the risks of medication. Failure to warn patients about side effects which might interfere with activities such as driving a vehicle or operating machinery have resulted in litigation.[24] Any failure to warn an outpatient about the soporific effects of any medication puts the psychiatrist at risk of liability. There has been one recorded case of failure to warn a patient using MAO inhibitors to refrain from eating foods containing tyramine.[25] The suit was not successful because the psychiatrist was able to prove that disclosure had been made. In the more recent literature there are reports of large out-of-court settlements for failure to warn patients taking neuroleptics of the risks of tardive dyskinesia.[26] This should not be surprising since tardive dyskinesia is a serious consequence of neuroleptic medicine, occurs with some frequency, and is a complication which develops slowly enough so that we have either been unaware of its dangers or have found it convenient not to frighten patients by mentioning the risk of its occurrence. It is conceivable that once a case involving tardive dyskinesia reaches a court of appeals and is decided in favor of the plaintiff that we will see many more suits in this area. Psychiatrists are understandably concerned about the malpractice implications of tardive dyskinesia. Most psychiatrists are still not warning patients or their families as to the full risk of this disorder. Recently a group of eminent researchers argued that writ-

[23]A. Stone, *Mental Health and Law: A System in Transition* (Rockville, Md.: DHEW, 1975), p. 105.

[24]Stone, *Mental Health and Law: A System in Transition.*

[25]"Medicolegal-Cheese and Tranylcypromine," *British Medical Journal* 3 (1970): 354.

[26]R. Sovner *et al.*, "Tardive Dyskinesia and Informed Consent," *Psychosomatics 19*, no. 3 (1978): 173.

ten rather than oral informed consent be obtained in two classes of
patients who are taking neuroleptics and who are at high risk of complications. These groups are, first, "Patients who have already developed
tardive dyskinesia, but who still require maintenance neuroleptic drug
therapy to prevent relapse of their psychiatric illness. There is a risk
among these patients that continued drug therapy may exacerbate the
severity of their abnormal movements or cause them to become irrever-
sible." The second group consists of patients who have received
neuroleptic drug therapy continuously for one year or more: "We consider patients to be at high risk for tardive dyskinesia after one year of
continuous treatment with neuroleptic agents."[27] These recommendations constitute a step forward in medical practice and in protecting
the physician. It is quite conceivable that they do not go far enough.
In the future we are very likely going to have to seek written consent for
the use of neuroleptics in many more situations than these researchers
have described.

Thus far the informed consent doctrine has not been applied to
group, individual, or family psychotherapy. It is the rare psychiatrist
who warns about the risks of psychotherapy. There is no record of any
practitioner's being sued for failing to do so. It is worthwhile, however,
for the psychiatrist to consider the reality that there are risks to
psychotherapy. Patients in any form of psychotherapy can get worse.
They can regress and become excessively dependent on the therapist or
they can be powerfully influenced in an adverse manner by the psychiatrist's values. These changes may be accompanied by a worsening of
symptoms. Patients in group therapy experience powerful pressures
toward conformity and a possible erosion of their sense of autonomy.
Family members who are not viewed as the identified patients often
agree to participate in family therapy to help their ailing relative and
immediately find that they too are treated like patients. They can become very upset during the course of family therapy. Yet they have not
only been uninformed as to this risk, but they have not even consented
to be patients. All patients who enter psychotherapy should be informed
as to risks regarding confidentiality. These risks (which will be discussed
in another section) are becoming increasingly serious.

Can the Patient Give Legal Consent without Signing a Consent Form?

No written form is required to make consent to treatment valid. The
patient's verbal consent is in effect a contract and most contracts are
made without a written record. From the standpoint of protecting him-

---

[27]*Ibid.*

self from malpractice suits, however, the psychiatrist is well advised to rely on written consent forms wherever possible. The written consent makes it possible to stipulate precisely what information has been provided to the patient. A patient who signs a consent form which lists all the possible risks of treatment cannot later claim that his consent was not informed.

Whether the patient has signed a consent form or merely gives oral consent, he is allowed to withdraw his consent at any time. The written consent form in no way affects the patient's right to change his mind and withdraw consent. This is sometimes an important issue with patients who have consented to receive ECT but who change their mind on the morning of treatment. Up until the brevitol is injected into the patient's vein, any statement made by the patient indicating he does not want treatment should be viewed as a withdrawal of consent.

What Malpractice Risks Are Involved in Treatment with Electroconvulsive Therapy?

Aside from informed consent issues which have already been discussed, the major suits related to the use of ECT have been based on negligence in use of premedication, negligence in post-ECT care, and negligent diagnosis and treatment of convulsion-related injuries.

When the use of muscle relaxants and sedatives as premedications was relatively new, one case arose around the issue of the physician's failure to utilize this form of premedication and subsequent harm to the patient in the form of a fracture.[28] Treatment in this case occurred in 1956 at a time when there were two schools of thought about ways of doing ECT and the suit was unsuccessful. Today, however, it would appear that providing ECT without premedication would be poor medical practice, and if the patient were harmed as a result of treatment the psychiatrist would probably be liable. It is also wise to monitor carefully the administration of drugs such as neuroleptics which have autonomic side effects and lower the seizure threshold. Patients should be kept on the lowest possible dosages of neuroleptics during the course of ECT.

Following ECT, patients are frequently confused and need to be carefully attended. There are several cases recorded in which patients were not watched carefully enough and sustained physical injuries as a result of their confusion.[29] Psychiatrists working in hospitals are held to an affirmative duty to monitor the patient and prevent self-injury when the patient is confused following the administration of shock therapy.

[28]Foxluger v. State, 23 Misc. 2d. 933, 203 N.Y.S.2d 985 (Ct. Cl. 1960).
[29]Brown v. Moore, 247 F.2d 711 (3d Cir. 1957); Meunier v. DePaul Hospital, 218 So. 2d 98 (La. Aff. 1969).

Failure to diagnose and treat fractures resulting from shock treatment is also actionable. It is important that psychiatrists be sensitive to the patient's complaints of pain and to other symptoms that might suggest fractures. Failure to order X rays to assist in the diagnostic process can be viewed as evidence of negligent diagnosis.[30]

With the increased efficiency of administration of ECT, suits involving physical injury have just about disappeared. The only future concern of the psychiatrist might be with regard to failure to inform the patient as to the possibility of loss of memory or impairment of other intellectual functions long after treatments are stopped. Competent psychiatrists always advise patients that a temporary organic brain syndrome will follow. There is much controversy in psychiatry, however, as to whether there is a risk of chronic "organicity." Certainly some patients do continue to complain of memory loss long after treatment. Most psychiatrists are unconvinced that such complaints are any more "organic" after treatment, but many still provide some warning that chronic memory loss can occur. Even if no information regarding this risk is given, the plaintiff would still have a difficult time proving the existence of damages. One patient has attempted to sue on an informed consent theory claiming memory loss after ECT, but the defendant argued effectively that her memory loss was due to a dissociative response and she was unsuccessful.[31]

What Are Some of the Risks of Malpractice in Using Pharmacotherapy?

The psychiatrist is in the same position as any physician who prescribes drugs. Failure to obtain informed consent puts him in jeopardy of liability. Use of inappropriate drugs, incompatible medications, or the wrong dosages can lead to lawsuits if the patient is harmed. While there are no recorded suits in psychiatric practice regarding using the wrong drug, the wrong dosage, or incompatible medications, this situation is very likely to change. This is one area of psychiatry in which standards of care can be enunciated relatively clearly. It is also an area in which errors are common.

Nonpsychiatric physicians are especially prone to make major errors in the use of psychotropic medications. Often, antianxiety drugs are prescribed for depression and antidepressives for anxiety. Powerful neuroleptics are often used to alleviate minor anxiety not associated with psychosis. There is a tendency to give small and ineffective dosages of tricyclics in treating depression. (In the past year I have seen two pa-

[30]Collins v. Hand, 431 Pa. 378, 246 A.2d (1968).
[31]Rice v. Nardini, Ca. 703-4, Docket no. 78N-1103 (D.C., 1976).

tients who were given a prescription for amitryptiline [elavil] by their physicians and told to take a pill whenever they were feeling depressed.) Quite commonly, both neuroleptic and antidepressant medications are prescribed in extremely low dosages and a therapeutic blood level is never obtained. It is conceivable that as laboratories become more skilled and efficient in determining blood levels of neuroleptics and antidepressants, psychiatrists using these drugs will be obligated to determine that the patient is receiving a therapeutic level of medication.

The psychiatrist who prescribes lithium is currently responsible for checking blood levels and ascertaining that toxic levels are not reached. Since lithium has relatively few adverse effects in therapeutic dosages but quite serious effects in excessive dosages, the psychiatrist is obligated to be alert to changes in blood levels which might herald toxic responses.

The psychiatrist is also obligated to ascertain that the patient is not receiving medications whose interactions might be harmful. If he prescribes MAOIs, for example, he must make certain that the patient is not using any adrenergic drugs such as ephedrine. It is also prudent to be familiar with the package insert or the *Physician's Desk Reference* statement as to any drug prescribed. These may be out of date, overly comprehensive, and overly conservative, but they might be used as standards in some cases and they do caution about all side effects and drug incompatibilities.

Psychiatrists who prescribe medication should be thoroughly familiar with the patient's physical condition. Many of the newer psychotropic medications have powerful effects on the body and their use may be contraindicated in a variety of physical conditions. The psychiatrist must either do a thorough history and examination himself or ascertain that a competent specialist has recently done so. Psychiatrists who engage primarily in office practice tend to be lax in evaluating the patient's physical condition. It is not too rare for a psychiatrist who is providing psychotherapy for a patient to offer the patient antidepressant medication when things are not going well. The physical examination may be deferred to avoid "laying hands" on the patient, and the psychiatrist may not be too diligent in making certain that the patient is examined by someone else. This is poor medical practice and legally risky.

What Are the Malpractice Risks for the Psychiatrist in Providing Psychotherapy?

There are only a few recorded cases in this area, all of which involve excessive intimacy with the patient. Except for situations in which there have been blatant violations of standard practice, the difficulties in proving negligent psychotherapy are formidable. It is difficult to assess psychological damages (which are the only damages likely to occur as a result of psychotherapy). It is even more difficult to develop proper standards for providing psychotherapy. There are dozens of schools of psychotherapy, each of which uses somewhat different techniques. A substantial minority of the profession can usually be found that will attest to the validity of almost any technique.

There has been much recent concern as to the ethical and legal implications of therapists' having sex with consenting patients. The psychiatrist who has sexual relations with a patient risks a malpractice suit as long as he continues to treat that patient and charge a fee. The helplessness of the psychiatric patient, the prolonged intimacy with her doctor, and the phenomenon of transference make the issue of seduction by a psychiatrist a more serious matter than seduction by a general physician. A nonpsychiatric physician who seduces hardly behaves in the tradition of Hypocrates, but it is unlikely that he is taking advantage of his patient in the same manner as a psychiatrist who behaves similarly.

Psychotherapy requires closeness between therapist and patient, and if it is to be successful the therapist must achieve that intimacy without using the patient to satisfy his own needs. In the course of achieving such closeness the patient develops powerful feelings for the therapist and is a relatively easy target for seduction. The therapist who has a sexual relationship with his patient may be satisfying some of the patient's needs, but he is also using the patient to satisfy his own needs. There is evidence that women who are seduced by male therapists are severely damaged by this experience, and often have considerable difficulty in benefiting from any subsequent therapeutic encounter. Even though they may not be visibly worsened by therapy it is probable that they are deprived of the opportunity of getting well. The situation is serious enough that the eminent sex researchers, Masters and Johnson, have argued that seduction of a patient by a psychiatrist should be viewed as a form of rape.[32]

The legal aspects of sexual seduction of patients raise interesting problems with regard to malpractice insurance. Some insurance companies have tried to argue that sexual seduction has nothing to do with medical practice and therefore cannot be negligent practice. Other insurance policies specifically exclude coverage for sexual involvement. Still others defend the physician as long as he denies the charges. (Obviously the patient's charges are not easily proved unless the physician

[32]W. H. Masters and V. E. Johnson, "Principles of the New Sex Therapy," *American Journal of Psychiatry* 133 (1976): 548–554.

admits having had sexual relations with the patient, unless several patients make the same accusation, or unless he has been moved to write love letters to the patient.) It is difficult to determine what current practices are, but it is likely that if claims are not too high most insurance companies seem to be settling these cases out of court.[33]

Some psychotherapists have publicly defended having sexual relationships with patients by calling such activity "treatment." They argue that patients are not harmed by such activities and may even be helped. It should be clear, however, that if the physician insists that sex was part of treatment and if the patient can prove that she was actually damaged by the psychotherapy experience (or prevented from obtaining necessary help), the suit is likely to be successful. In at least one case the insurer was unable to avoid the obligation to pay damages when the physician insisted his sexual involvement was therapeutic. It seems possible that his claim was such as to put the entire issue into a treatment perspective and to define the issue as one involving malpractice.[34]

Punitive sanctions other than lawsuits can be invoked when psychiatrists have sexual relationships with their patients. There are cases in which therapists have had their licenses to practice medicine revoked for having sexual intercourse with consenting patients.[35] It has been much more difficult to dismiss defending psychiatrists from professional organizations since these organizations have not as a rule created a legal structure which would enable them to enforce such action.

It is not uncommon these days for therapist and patient to fall in love and desire physical intimacies with one another. The physician who has consenting physical relations with a patient is in no legal jeopardy unless he does so while continuing to treat and bill her as a patient. In those instances where a therapist finds both he and his patient desire to be lovers rather than therapist and patient, he should terminate the professional relationship and find his patient a new therapist.

I have discussed sexual relations between patient and therapist in terms of a male therapist and female patient. All the current literature focuses on this type of pairing. As more women become psychiatrists, however, we may also see lawsuits brought by male patients who claim seduction. With greater acknowledgment and acceptance of homosexuality in our society, we may also see suits claiming homosexual seduction.

For the moment at least, it would seem that the ethical psychiatrist

---

[33]A. Stone, "Legal Implications of Sexual Activities Between Psychiatrists and Patients," *American Journal of Psychiatry 133* (1976): 1138–41.
[34]Keiser v. Berry, Cir. Ct. 78-8182 (Fla. 1979).
[35]Stone, "Legal Implications of Sexual Activities."

is in little danger of malpractice suits related to psychotherapy. As long as the transference is not exploited and the patient is not physically or sexually abused, it is hard to see how the psychiatrist could be successfully sued even if the results of therapy are horrendous. It is the psychotherapist's near immunity to lawsuits which has prompted a renewed interest in applying the theories of contract and strict liability to psychiatric practice.

Is the Psychiatrist Responsible for Initiating Care of his Patients When They Develop Nonpsychiatric Illnesses?

The answer here is obviously yes. This question is included primarily to remind the psychiatrist that the patient's physical complaints cannot be ignored. When a psychiatrist hears complaints suggestive of physical disturbance from his outpatient, he must either investigate and treat the patient or ascertain that someone else does. In the hospital setting the psychiatrist is responsible for diagnosing and treating any current physical illnesses. Evaluating the bizarre and sometimes esoteric physical complaints of a patient who is known to be hysterical or psychotic can be tedious. Psychiatrists must remember, however, that the mentally ill can develop nonpsychiatric illnesses just as easily as anyone else.

To What Extent Is the Psychiatrist Liable for the Negligent Practice of Other Professionals?

Under the theory of vicarious liability, the doctor is usually liable for the negligence of somebody he directly employs. A doctor who employs a nurse or technician assumes a liability for that person's professional conduct. Relatively few psychiatrists employ nurses or technicians, however, and the major concern of psychiatrists in this area involves liability for the negligence of other physicians. If one professional employs another, their relationship may be viewed as a master–servant relationship with the employer being responsible for the negligence of the employee. The situation in medicine, however, is somewhat different from that in other professions. Because of the discretion, judgment, and freedom of action that is inherent in the practice of medicine, the employed physician might be classified as an "independent contractor" rather than a servant. The existence of some economic relationship between two physicians does not automatically create a master–servant relationship, and vicarious liability does not always hold.[36]

Psychiatrists must always be concerned with the negligence of interns and residents. Although these physicians are usually employed by the hospital, they do work under the supervision of the attending psychiatrist and are sometimes viewed as "borrowed servants." The attending physician may be liable for their negligence if he is derelict in supervising them or if he assigns them responsibilities that are beyond their ability or level of training. The attending physician may also be liable if he fails to see his patients periodically and entrusts them totally to a trainee who makes a mistake in diagnosis or treatment.[37]

The borrowed servant and vicarious liability doctrines are declining in usage. They originated at a time when large charitable or government hospitals were granted immunity from virtually all tort liability, including that based on culpable actions of hospital employees. By imposing vicarious liability on the attending physician, the courts hoped to assure that injured parties would have at least one solvent defendant against whom to proceed. As hospitals have become less immune to liability and as physicians at all levels of training, including interns and residents, have insured themselves against malpractice, the doctrine of vicarious liability has made less sense. Psychiatrists still retain an obligation to provide duly careful supervision of all doctors who work under them. But there is a new tendency to bring suits, arising out of the negligent actions of interns or residents, against the hospital rather than against the attending physician.[38]

What Are the Psychiatrist's Obligations When the Patient Wishes to Terminate Treatment?

Ideally, the patient who asks to terminate the physician–patient relationship will have made sufficient improvement so no further treatment is needed. If the psychiatrist concurs with the patient's decision to terminate treatment, this is a happy situation and there is no legal problem. The patient, however, may want to terminate before the doctor thinks he is ready. Here the psychiatrist is obligated to warn patients as to the risks of terminating therapy. If the patient continues to insist on termination, the psychiatrist would be well advised to urge the patient

[36]A. R. Holder, *Medical Malpractice Law* (New York: Wiley, 1975), p. 216.
[37]*Ibid.*, p. 202.
[38]Annas, *Rights of Hospital Patients*, p. 57.

to find another doctor who might continue treatment. The psychiatrist would then be required to provide full information as to the patient's previous treatment to the new doctor. It is prudent to ask patients with serious emotional disturbances, whether they be outpatients or inpatients, to sign a form stating that they are leaving treatment against medical advice whenever the doctor feels that termination is unwise. If the patient refuses to sign such a form, a note should be put in the chart documenting that termination of the relationship is against the doctor's advice.

What Legal Issues Are Involved When the Physician Terminates Treatment?

There are a number of reasons why a psychiatrist might want to terminate a professional relationship with a patient. The least honorable reason is that the patient cannot pay his bills. Unfortunately, there are therapists who will stop treatment of those who become impecunious in the course of therapy. There are other reasons for the doctor's terminating the relationship which have greater ethical justification. In a psychotherapy relationship, transference and countertransference feelings may get out of hand. The doctor may become convinced that the patient would do better with a different therapist. Or the patient may manifest an unwillingness to cooperate in the treatment process. Sometimes the doctor becomes convinced that the patient would do better without treatment and that the patient's continuation of treatment is based on exaggerated dependency wishes or even an effort to justify inactivity. It is not unheard of for patients to want to remain in therapy to avoid responsibility, to gain power in social systems, and to avoid criminal sanction.

In all of the above situations, the physician can terminate the relationship if he provides the patient with reasonable notice of his intention to terminate, gives the patient reasonable time to find a new doctor, assists in that process, and provides his records to the new doctor.[39] The situation is somewhat thornier when the psychiatrist honestly believes that the patient would be better off without any kind of continued therapy at all but knows that the patient wants to continue therapy. In this instance, it would seem useful for the psychiatrist to explain that a holiday from therapy might be most desirable, but still to give the patient time to find another doctor if the patient insists on the need for further treatment.

[39]Holder, *Medical Malpractice Law*, chap. 12.

The physician can never unilaterally sever a professional relationship with a patient when there is still a need for continuing medical attention without giving the patient reasonable notice and assisting the patient in obtaining continued care. If a physician does this, he is liable under the doctrine of abandonment.[40] Abandonment may occur through direct and explicit withdrawal from the case or through less overt behavior such as continued failure to attend a patient.

Psychiatrists tend to be somewhat more cavalier than other medical practitioners in terminating treatment. This may be because of the more elective nature of certain interventions such as psychotherapy. Or it may be related to difficulties encountered in treating emotionally disturbed people who often have abrasive personality traits. There are probably many terminations of treatment related to the patient's financial situation or to his abrasive personality traits which cannot be justified ethically. They cannot be justified legally either if the psychiatrist simply announces to the patient that treatment will be terminated and makes no effort to explain the reasons for this decision or to give the patient ample time to deal with the consequences of termination.

Psychiatrists also have a tendency (as do all mental health practitioners) to tell certain patients that they need treatment, but then to tell them that they will have to see another therapist who is less busy or has cheaper rates. There is nothing illegal about this. One of the few rights the doctor does have is the right in nonemergency situations to select his patients. But it is not uncommon for highly disturbed patients to be rejected by several therapists and be put on psychotherapy waiting lists while their condition deteriorates. Our profession and mental health agencies have a moral obligation to see that this does not happen. If we do not find ways of resolving this type of problem, our obligation may become legal as well as moral.

[40]*Ibid.*

PART II

THE REGULATION OF PSYCHIATRIC PRACTICE BY LEGISLATIVE BODIES AND THE COURTS

Although psychiatric practice is certainly influenced by the deterrent aspects of malpractice law, psychiatrists should not find the general use of this form of regulation oppressive. In the great majority of instances a successful malpractice suit is based on substantial evidence that the doctor has done something wrong and that the patient has been harmed. Medical societies cannot always impose sanctions on members who take advantage of patients or who practice sloppily. Malpractice law, by providing such sanctions, helps to demarcate the boundary between good and bad medical practice.

In most instances successful malpractice suits punish only errant practitioners. The profession as a whole is not directly affected. Only an occasional ruling coming from a higher court of appeal has broad or sweeping consequences which may affect all practitioners. And even decisions which seem to be directed at the profession as a whole may not have as global an influence as we fear. Most psychiatrists, for example, initially feared that the *Tarasoff* ruling would impose an unfair responsibility and burden on all members of our profession. But even this highly controversial ruling was based on a set of unusual circumstances which are not likely to recur with sufficient frequency so as to influence the majority of practitioners.

It is something totally different when statutes or federal court decisions place definite limits on what all psychiatrists can or cannot do in the course of daily treatment of patients. This is direct regulation of psychiatric practice, and the psychiatrist's intentions, good or bad, or his competence are not relevant. Rather, all psychiatrists from the best to the worst are required by statute or by court order to behave in a certain manner, and if they fail to do so they violate the law. There is, of course, no problem when statutes or court orders require behavior on the part of psychiatrists that is consistent with good medical practice. There is a problem, however, if psychiatrists perceive some of the recent statutes and court rulings as so restrictive as to interfere with good medical practice or even to prevent it. It is natural that we perceive as offensive legal regulation which diminishes our power to decide what is best for the patient. It is natural that we perceive as oppressive legal restraint on our freedom to practice medicine in accordance with our conscience and skills.

Most of the legal restrictiveness psychiatrists are currently experiencing involves our relationship with highly disturbed patients who resist psychiatric treatment. In an effort to assure that the civil liberties of resistant patients are not compromised, the legislatures and the courts have imposed substantial limitations on the role of the psychiatrist in the civil commitment process. They have provided guidelines as to what kinds of treatment can and cannot be used in specific situations, and have attempted to mandate standards of treatment. Here, there is a clear difference in the process of regulation of psychiatric treatment by tort law as opposed to its regulation by court order or statute. The standards for what is acceptable medical practice in malpractice law are defined by the medical profession. In statutory and judicial rulings involving the care of many severely disturbed patients, they are defined by courts and legislators. Much of what the psychiatrist now can or cannot do is determined by law. It is, therefore, no longer possible to treat severely disturbed patients without awareness and knowledge of that law.

The main issues which will be considered in Part II will be involuntary commitment to mental hospitals and the rights of patients in the commitment process, including the patient's right to treatment and his right to refuse treatment. Some effort will be made to deal with the extremely elusive issue of competency, specifically the patient's competency to refuse or accept treatment. The impact of new legal restraints on the psychiatric treatment of children will be reviewed briefly.

The behavior of psychiatrists with regard to the issue of confidentiality is regulated by statutes, malpractice decisions, and federal agencies. Malpractice issues related to confidentiality have already been discussed in Part I. Other issues regarding confidentiality will be discussed at the end of this section.

7

Civil Commitment

It is difficult to discuss the issue of the involuntary commitment and treatment of severely disturbed patients dispassionately. Some argue that it is immoral to deprive almost any noncriminal person of freedom. Others believe it is immoral to fail to treat sick people even when they say they do not want treatment. Conflicts between the values of freedom and the values of health and compassion are powerful, and most commentators in this area take relatively unyielding positions on one or the other side of this dispute. Papers and books published in this area tend to resemble polemics or legal briefs more than scientific treatises. It is common for writers to cite only studies that support their argument and to ignore all others. Even more or less official documents such as the "Model Code" for civil commitment prepared by the American Bar Association Commission on the Mentally Disabled and the American Civil Liberties Union handbook *The Rights of Mental Patients* take an open adversarial stance in supporting freedom values over health values.[1]

Conceptual Biases

As a practicing psychiatrist, it would be extremely difficult for me to discuss the issues involved in involuntary treatment of the severely disturbed patient in an unbiased manner. I have strong beliefs about these issues which will influence the manner in which I present information and conceptualize issues. The reader may find it easier to deal with my biases if these are stated openly before specific problem areas are considered. My opinions can be briefly summarized as follows:

1. *Mental illness exists.* There are a group of behavior disorders

[1] B. J. Ennis and R. D. Emery, *The Rights of Mental Patients* (New York: Avon, 1978); Commission on the Mentally Disabled, American Bar Association, "Suggested Statute on Civil Commitment," *Mental Disability Law Reporter 2*, no. 1 (1977).

which for scientific and humanistic as well as for pragmatic reasons are appropriately considered under an illness model. Many of the behavior disorders which psychiatrists treat are based on documented organic dysfunction and these disorders are illnesses in the same sense that any physical disorders are illnesses. In other disorders we call mental illnesses the similarities to physical illness are not always so apparent, but a strong case can still be made for considering the most severe disturbances under an illness model.

2. *A patient who has a severe mental illness experiences profound suffering.* The anguish of severe mental illness is no less than that associated with severe physical illness. Mental illness can lead to total disability, a life of continuous agony and death.

3. *Many severe mental illnesses are treatable.* In the majority of cases, treatment does not totally cure the disturbance but mitigates its more malignant aspects by relieving painful symptoms, enabling the patient to function more efficiently. Attorneys often have difficulty in appreciating that the psychiatrists' inability to cure most of their patients does not distinguish psychiatric practice from other types of medical practice. Many if not most medical illnesses are not curable but are, rather, modifiable. The likelihood that patients will not be cured by psychiatric treatment does not mean that such intervention is worthless, nor does it in itself constitute an argument for restricting such treatment.

4. *Severe mental illness is manifested by disorders of thinking, of emotionality, and of decision-making capability.* Some behavior disorders are clearly caused by brain malfunction and the majority are probably associated with some type of brain malfunction. The person who is mentally ill cannot always make judgments as to the risks and benefits of a given treatment in a manner which serves his own interests. Stated differently, a person who is mentally ill may not be able to decide what is best for himself. The "best for himself" in this instance would refer to what the patient might have decided if he were not mentally ill. (Or if an objective standard is preferred, it might refer to what the "reasonable man" would choose.)

Civil liberties attorneys have been quick to point out the danger of circularity in this kind of reasoning and the possibility that people who do not accept the doctor's recommendations as to what is best for them are in jeopardy of having their refusal interpreted as a sign of their illness.[2] Certainly, circular thinking and viewing efforts to resist treatment as signs of illness are not unknown in psychiatry. But the possibility of sloppy thinking about a patient's refusal to accept treatment

---

[2]B. J. Ennis, *Prisoners of Psychiatry: Mental Patients, Psychiatrists and the Law* (New York: Harcourt Brace Jovanovich, 1972).

should not be used to distract anyone from dealing with the reality that a person with impaired brain functioning may not be able accurately to perceive and assess the risks and benefits of treatment.

It is easiest to illustrate how disease can produce incompetent judgment by visualizing a situation in which a patient has contacted a severe bacterial pneumonia, is running a temperature of 105°, and is delirious. The patient will almost certainly be cured if he receives antibiotic therapy and will almost certainly die if he does not. In his delirious state the patient believes that the doctor who wishes to give him an injection of penicillin is trying to hurt him, and he refuses to take the medicine.

I believe that in this situation the patient does not know what is best for him and the doctor does. It is also clear that only the most insensitive and incompetent physician would fail to search for any possible means of treating that patient involuntarily. Note that this argument can be expanded to justify involuntary hospitalization. If the patient needed oxygen and continued nursing care, hospitalization would be as integral a part of treatment as antibiotic medication. The moral case for hospitalization which might restrict the patient's freedom would be just as strong as the moral case for involuntary antibiotic treatment.

Hopefully, even the most rabid believer in always adhering to the patient's verbalized wishes would appreciate the absurdity of honoring the patient's wishes in this extreme situation. But there are many other less obvious situations in which honoring the patient's verbalized wishes is equally absurd. Patients whose sensoria are clouded because of a variety of organic brain syndromes often cannot make decisions in their best interests. It is also unlikely that the manic patient who has been agitated and who has not slept for five days could make a rational risk–benefit assessment of whether treatment would be in his own best interests. Nor could the psychotically depressed individual who believes that he has sinned unforgivably and deserves to die be expected to make a self-serving judgment as to whether to accept or refuse treatment.

Perhaps because Americans are so committed to the value of personal autonomy and so fearful of political oppression, we are especially offended by the idea that someone else could ever know what is best for any individual. Some libertarian zealots will never concede that there are times when an individual's best interests dictate that he be controlled by others. Yet such a belief can be maintained only by denying the limits of human potentiality and the realities of human vulnerability. There are times in the lives of most people when their judgment is severely impaired because of illness and when they are better off relying on the judgment of others. The reality that people with severe illnesses may have impaired capacity to determine whether various interventions are in their own best interests is an essential justification of involuntary treatment. It is difficult to justify hospitalizing and treating people involuntarily unless we believe that their decision-making capacities are impaired.

5. *Hospitalization leads to serious infringement of the patient's liberties.* There are side effects to hospitalization such as learned dependency, institutionalization, regression, and stigmatization which may leave the patient worse off than he was before being hospitalized.[3] As has been noted in the section on malpractice, many psychiatric treatments may also have serious harmful consequences to the patient. The process of involuntary hospitalization and involuntary treatment must therefore be carefully monitored. The patient and society must have some assurance that hospitalization can be helpful to the patient. This means that there must be treatments available to the committed patient which will have a substantial likelihood of alleviating his symptoms. A society committed to humanistic and compassionate treatment of the mentally ill should not accept the practice of involuntary confinement if no treatment is available. It should not accept hospitalization followed by interventions which do nothing but control the patient's activity within the institution. It should not tolerate treatment that harms the patient more than it helps him.

Because patients can be harmed by involuntary commitment and involuntary treatment, it is essential that these activities be monitored by the courts. Decisions regarding involuntary intervention have a moral as well as a medical component. It is unfair to the patient and to the doctor to leave the decision as to commitment and treatment entirely up to the doctor. The courts must know when involuntary treatment is being considered and must have control over its use.

6. *Treatment in many of our mental hospitals is inadequate.* For some involuntarily hospitalized patients, the end result of treatment and commitment may be worse than no commitment and no treatment. It is also true, however, that hospitalization can be helpful to many patients and that the benefits can be maximized and the harms minimized by improving the quality of care provided to patients. In a hospital which is adequately funded and adequately staffed, the benefits of involuntary treatment are likely to outweigh the risks. Most of the arguments against involuntary commitment would have little relevance if all hospitals gave excellent care.

The above observations suggest that there are two major ways of preventing harm to patients who are likely to be hospitalized and treated involuntarily. The first and most obvious way is to improve the condi-

[3]S. L. Halleck, *The Politics of Therapy* (New York: Science House, 1971).

tion of mental hospitals. This, of course, is an expensive alternative. It is also likely to be unpopular. As a rule, the public and its elected representatives invest money in mental health programs grudgingly. The mentally ill are not a particularly attractive or influential voting bloc. A second way in which our society can protect patients from harm as a result of inadequate hospital care is simply to keep them out of hospitals. This, of course, has been the protective strategy advocated by civil liberties attorneys. They have had great success in the courts and with legislators in shaping a series of decisions and laws which substantially restrict the population of patients who can be involuntarily committed to a mental hospital. (In fairness, it should be noted that some civil-liberties-inspired lawsuits have been designed to improve the conditions of mental hospitals. The success of these suits and the probable motives of their advocates will be discussed later.) Strategies of mental health care which involve keeping people out of the hospital through any means, including legal action, have widespread public appeal. Nobody wants to see people hospitalized unnecessarily. Those who believe strongly in the merits of community treatment sometimes welcome any actions that keep the people in the community. Those libertarians who believe that freedom values are more important than all others will welcome any actions that make it difficult to restrict anyone's liberty. Those taxpayers who are totally unconcerned with the plight of people less fortunate than themselves welcome the perceived opportunity of saving money.

One factor that has guided civil liberties advocates in opting for the solution of keeping patients out of hospitals has been their sincere belief that highly disturbed patients could be more effectively treated in the community. Unfortunately, there is no assurance that people who are kept out of mental hospitals receive decent treatment. The development of community resources for severely disturbed people has not proceeded in an efficient or encouraging manner in the last decade. Even when resources have been available, they have often been poorly utilized by patients too disturbed to accept them. Yet as a result of the new laws, extremely disturbed patients must find some means of surviving in highly stressful communities. Not surprisingly, the crusade to liberate patients from the hospital and treat them in the community has had equivocal and sometimes tragic results. Tens of thousands of mental patients now live outside hospitals in conditions of neglect and misery which make their lives every bit as dreadful as they were in the worst of mental hospitals.[4]

In summary, the decision to deal with bad treatment in hospitals by

[4]R. Reich and L. Siegel, "The Chronically Mentally Ill Shuffle to Oblivion," *Psychiatric Annals 5*, no. 4 (1975).

restricting treatment rather than by improving it was extremely ill-advised and has worsened the plight of the mentally ill.

7. *The major strategy by which our courts and legislators have elected to restrict the process of involuntary commitment has involved efforts to provide patients with the same legal rights as have traditionally been provided to those accused of criminal acts.* A patient who faces commitment now has a number of new rights. These rights have radically altered many aspects of the civil commitment process, but their most powerful influence is apparent in the development of new standards for commitment. As the courts have sought to protect mental patients, the standards of commitments were changed to provide "objective" criteria by which the courts could make commitment decisions without having to rely on the "subjective" opinions of doctors.[5] We have now moved from a standard for commitment which merely requires a diagnosis of mental illness and need for treatment to one which requires an additional finding that the patient is dangerous to himself or others. The "dangerousness" standard is now part of statutory law in many states and has been heavily supported by higher federal courts and indirectly by the Supreme Court.[6]

I believe that the imposition of the "dangerousness" standard on the commitment process diminishes the possibility of providing humane or effective treatment for the mentally ill. Reliance on that standard is keeping severely disturbed but treatable patients out of hospitals. At the same time it is filling our hospitals with highly disturbed and highly destructive individuals who probably cannot be treated. While many of the new rights afforded patients are desirable, it is doubtful that handling the commitment procedure like a criminal proceeding, and in particular relying on a standard of dangerousness, can ultimately be anything but harmful to patients and destructive to the morale of those who must care for these patients.

Reliance on the criminal justice model in dealing with the mentally ill is also expensive. The growing number of attorneys who must be employed to deal with issues litigated through criminal justice processes and the accompanying drain on medical staff time may ultimately lead to public expenditures which are far greater than would have been required to bring our hospitals up to decent standards.

8. *It is possible to devise ways of hospitalizing and treating people on an involuntary basis so that, in proper balance, the values of freedom, health, and compassion can be served at the same time.* This would require that patients retain most of the due process rights they now have. It would require

---

[5]Ennis and Emery, *Rights of Mental Patients*, chap. 2.
[6]A. Stone, *Mental Health and Law: A System in Transition* (Rockville, Md.: NIMH, 1975); T. Szasz, *Psychiatric Slavery* (New York: The Free Press, 1977).

the elimination of the "dangerousness" standard. It would require that commitment be based only on the following criteria: (a) the presence of a severe mental illness; (b) the availability of a treatment for that illness; and (c) a determination that the patient is not competent to make a rational appraisal of his need for treatment.

9. *It is essential that the issues of involuntary hospitalization and involuntary treatment not be separated.* Hospitalization is only one form of treatment. Under current laws we are now encountering situations in which people are deprived of freedom but still have a right to refuse treatment which might make them well. Patients who lack the capacity to make rational decisions as to their need for hospitalization also lack the capacity to make decisions as to their need for various treatments. The issue of involuntary hospitalization and involuntary treatment with interventions other than hospitalization are really the same issue. They should be resolved at the same judicial hearing so that a patient who is involuntarily hospitalized is automatically defined as a patient who cannot refuse other forms of treatment.

The above opinions will obviously color much of the following discussion. Some of the positions I have taken are presented in editorial form and are not supported by argument or data. To those unfamiliar with the issues, my statements may be perceived as mere polemics. (Of course, all writing in this area is polemical. No one has ever studied the result of involuntary commitment on patients in a serious way.) In the ensuing part of this section, I will present material which I hope will clarify why I take the above positions.

What Are the Major Recent Changes Regarding Legal Regulation of Treatment of Severe Illness?

Most of the changes which influence psychiatric practice have been the result of court decisions and legislation made in the last ten years. Only a few years ago psychiatrists in most states had enormous power to initiate commitment of patients to restrain them and to treat them without judicial intervention. Even when the final determination of civil commitment was made by the courts, the psychiatrist's opinion was almost never questioned. In some states commitment was simply based on medical certification by two or more physicians. The certification was not reviewed by the courts but by an administrative board or commission comprised partially of physicians. Here again it was rare for the doctor's recommendation to be ignored. There was little the patient could do to avoid commitment once the doctor had formally stated that the patient was mentally ill and in need of treatment. Judicial hearings tended to be perfunctory; sometimes the patient was not even notified of the hearing. Often the patient was not present at the hearing, and it was extremely rare for the patient to employ the services of an attorney in resisting commitment. The standards for commitment were vague and based largely on the doctor's opinion regarding the presence of illness and the need for treatment.[7]

Until only a few years ago, psychiatrists did not have to worry about patients' refusing treatment. Since patients were easily committed and the committed patient was usually viewed as incompetent, treatment was given whether the patient agreed to it or not. Often the consent of the family was sought when a patient resisted treatment, and it was usually assumed that this substitute consent was sufficient legally to override any of the patient's objections.

If a psychiatrist had for some reason been out of touch with the realities of psychiatric practice for the last ten years (let us assume he had been on a prolonged voyage) and then returned to practice, he might perceive himself as having returned to a new world. Dangerousness to self or others has now become a necessary standard for commitment in most states. A majority of states now require a judicial hearing for nonemergency commitments. Efforts are routinely made to provide all people facing civil commitment with most of the same legal protections provided to those accused of crimes. In the majority of states patients facing civil commitment are entitled to their own or court-appointed attorneys. It is now more likely that not that a patient who vigorously opposes commitment will not be hospitalized. The decision-making power with regard to civil commitment has shifted decisively from the medical to the legal profession. *Psychiatrists who have become sophisticated in working in this area no longer speak of committing a patient; rather, they speak of initiating a petition for commitment or of assisting the court in the commitment process.* This new manner of addressing the issue accurately reflects current reality. In theory it may never have been true that the psychiatrist committed patients. In past decades, however, the psychiatrist was in a "de facto" sense the person who committed patients. Today there is no ambiguity on this issue. It is only the court that can commit, and the psychiatrist's role in the commitment process is primarily that of assisting the court. A psychiatrist returning from a prolonged voyage would also be shocked to find that he had little freedom to treat even the most disturbed patients who do not consent to treatment. He would find that in some states courts had imposed standards for treatment and that in most states certain treatments such as

[7]American Bar Foundation, *The Mentally Disabled and the Law* (Washington, D.C.: ABF, 1971), pp. 1–8.

electroconvulsive therapy could not be given to nonconsenting patients unless efforts were made to obtain a guardianship for the patient.

Bruce Ennis, the legal director of the American Civil Liberties Union, has noted that the law regarding rights of mental patients has changed faster than any other area of law.[8] He notes that in only the last five years a very substantial body of mental health case law has developed and in that same time a very large and growing mental health bar has emerged. In effect, a new specialty of law involving mentally disordered patients has developed. Attorneys now have a substantial and often critical influence in shaping the destiny of the mentally ill.

What Speculations Can Be Made as to Why the Above Changes Have Developed?

It is much too early to gain a scholarly perspective on the many factors that have contributed to the emergence of the new legal regulation of psychiatric care. It is possible to speculate as to why we have experienced so much change, and in my opinion the following factors are important:

1. During the 1960s our society developed an expanded awareness of the oppression of minorities and a powerful commitment to preserving the rights of minorities. The most powerful thrust of the civil rights movement was toward protecting the rights of black people, but the movement spread quickly to support many other minorities such as youth, criminals, the elderly, and the mentally disordered. The electronic media, particularly television, played an important role in increasing public awareness of oppressive situations, including conditions existing in mental hospitals.
2. The level of care provided to patients in some of the larger public mental health hospitals was certainly poor during the 1960s and in no sense comparable to the level of care provided in private hospitals. Many patients were hospitalized unnecessarily and were put into situations where they received inadequate treatment. The new legal approach to the problem of mental dysfunction did serve to alleviate a certain amount of oppressiveness inflicted upon the mentally ill. It was warmly received by a civil-rights-minded society.
3. The psychiatric profession was not resistant to changing the

[8]Ennis and Emery, *Rights of Mental Patients*, p. 13.

mental health system and often welcomed change. Many of us were deeply troubled when we observed what was happening to some mentally ill patients, and we hoped that expanding their rights would not only protect them, but would lead to development of a superior system of mental health care. Some psychiatrists, including myself, even viewed the emphasis on dangerousness as a desirable change in the criteria for commitment.[9] Those of us who welcomed the new effort to protect the rights of the mentally ill failed to foresee the extent to which it would lead to so much legal regulation of medical treatment.

4. The legal changes involving the mental health system were catalyzed by the efforts of a group of exceptionally dedicated and brilliant young attorneys, associated with the American Civil Liberties Union and the Mental Health Law Project. As a rule attorneys for the defendants or the state could not match the reform lawyers in degree of commitment, available time, or available resources. The reform-minded lawyers were quite frank, and are still quite frank, in stating that their primary objective was to abolish civil commitment.[10] Sensing that they were unlikely to obtain this goal, however, they were adept at compromising and adapted a strategy designed to restrict involuntary commitment by expanding the rights of patients or by obtaining court rulings which made it difficult for hospitals to retain patients in settings which provided inadequate treatment. In adopting the tactic of providing the mental patient the same rights as the criminal, the reform movement created an urgent need for attorneys familiar with mental health issues. A mental health bar was created and it grew rapidly. The existence of this bar in itself now constitutes a vested interest toward maintaining a status quo in which legal regulation of commitment and treatment will continue. Ironically, however, if this bar is to sustain itself it will also serve as a powerful resistance to abolishment of civil commitment.

5. The political climate of the 1970s ideally suited a move toward expanding the freedom of psychiatric patients and spending as little as possible to improve their plight. This was a time when taxpayers were reluctant to spend money on disadvantaged citizens. It was an era in which our society developed a powerful commitment to the value of freedom but showed diminishing commitment to the value of compassion. A legalistic approach to

---

[9]S. L. Halleck, "The Psychiatrist and the Legal Process," *Psychology Today*, February 1969.
[10]Ennis and Emery, *Rights of Mental Patients*, Chap. 2.

the problem of mental illness tends to camouflage its dimensions. Those who wished to avoid facing the realities of the suffering of the mentally ill, those who were passionately committed to the value of freedom, and those who had no motivation but to save money, were all able to join together in supporting legalization of the commitment and treatment process.

What Are Some of the Mechanisms by Which the New Legal Approach to the Treatment of Mental Disorders Has Been Instituted?

Most of the recent changes have been brought about through the federal courts. Patients have brought actions on their own behalf or on the behalf of other persons similarly situated (class-action suits) to have certain restrictions put on them declared unconstitutional. In a few instances the plaintiffs have cited statutory law in support of their case, but for the most part they have won their cases by successfully pleading that various actions taken by the mental health system deprived them of their constitutional rights as guaranteed by the First, Eighth, and Fourteenth Amendments.[11]

In most instances in which change is initiated, higher federal courts first rule that existing practices regarding certain aspects of involuntary commitment are unconstitutional. State legislatures then respond to these rulings by devising new statutes regarding treatment of the mentally disabled which meet the constitutional requirements imposed by the courts. The above process is time-consuming and complex. In many of the critical cases, lower courts initially ruled against the plaintiffs but were overruled on appeal to higher courts. Some of the major cases which served as landmarks or precedents for other cases are still being appealed. Even though a case is being appealed, however, it may still influence psychiatric practice. In the process of appeal a court may issue an injunction or writ which prohibits state mental health professionals from treating patients in a way which is in the process of being contested.

Some of the most important suits have been supported by an old federal statute under Title 42 of the U.S. Code, section 1983, which states: "every person who under color of any statute, ordinance, regulation, custom, or usage, of any state or territory, who subjects or causes to be subjected any citizen of the United States or other person within the jurisdiction thereof the deprivation of any rights, privileges, or im-

[11]Lessard v. Schmidt, 349 F. Supp. 1078 (E.D. Wis., 1972); Hawks v. Lazaro, 202 S.E.2d 109 (W.Va. 1974); Suzuki v. Quisenberry, 411 F. Supp. 1113 (D. Ha. 1976).

munities secured by the constitution and laws shall be liable to the parties injured in an action in law, suit in equity, or other proper proceeding for redress." In effect, the above-quoted "1983 Statute" makes it possible to sue doctors for damages even when the doctor is obeying the law. The weapon of a federally sanctioned suit for damages against doctors and mental health officials has served as an important adjunct or wedge for civil liberties lawyers seeking to expand patient's rights. [12]

Once the courts accept the argument that deprivation of liberty of a person who is mentally ill is substantially the same as deprivation of liberty imposed upon the criminal, the argument for changing the mental health system in the direction of providing greater legal protection for patients follows ineluctably. The major cases in this area have been well articulated, well reasoned, and effectively argued. The medical profession and psychiatric organizations have been relatively passive and unwilling to adapt adversarial strategies for controlling the extent of change. It is only quite recently that psychiatrists and attorneys employed by psychiatric organizations have begun to contest certain aspects of change.

Given the Recent Changes, What Are the Psychiatrist's Current Roles in the Commitment Process?

Although most of the major legal issues in civil commitment have not yet been discussed, their relevance to psychiatric practice may be better understood if the current roles of the psychiatrist are first explained. (It should be emphasized that the psychiatrist's role will vary from state to state. What are described here are roles that are fairly typical.) There are several kinds of situations in which the psychiatrist might find himself assisting in the commitment process. Psychiatrists working in emergency rooms, or seeing a patient in a clinic or a private office, may feel that a particular patient desperately needs hospitalization. The patient may refuse hospitalization. If the psychiatrist then feels that the patient meets the standards for commitment (usually, that he is dangerous to himself or others and mentally ill or inebriate), the psychiatrist can either urge the patient's family or friends to initiate a petition to commit the patient or the psychiatrist can himself serve as the petitioner who initiates commitment. Where the psychiatrist is the petitioner he must fill out the proper forms himself. The decision to

---

[12]A. Stone, "The Commission on Judicial Action of the American Psychiatric Association: Origins and Prospects—A Personal View," *Bulletin of the American Academy of Psychiatry and the Law 3*, no. 3 (1975): 119.

petition for involuntary commitment is always a judgment issue for the psychiatrist. He is not obligated by law to petition for commitment or to urge others to petition. If he does initiate commitment he takes little risk of liability for breach of confidentiality in this process, nor is he likely to be sued for false imprisonment unless his petition is based on intentions that might be harmful to the patient.

Once a petition for commitment has been received by an officer of the court (a clerk or magistrate) the patient is usually ordered to be examined, either at a mental health center or hospital. This examination follows shortly, usually within twenty-four hours of the receipt of the petition by the court. A second way in which a psychiatrist can become involved in the commitment process is by serving as an official examiner, either at a mental health center or a psychiatric hospital. (The psychiatrist at this stage of the commitment process is an agent of the court and in many states is provided with immunity from lawsuits.) As an official examiner the psychiatrist will be asked to make a determination as to whether or not the patient meets the criteria for involuntary commitment and to pass this information on to the court by completing the proper forms. Psychiatrists who work in hospitals which treat committed patients might in emergency situations serve in the role of petitioner and official examiner at the same time. Once the examining psychiatrist has recommended commitment and the magistrate has approved it, the patient is usually taken to a hospital ward designated as a unit that accepts committed patients. Here the hospital-employed psychiatrist may also be required to report to the court as to whether or not the patient meets the criteria for commitment.

A final way in which a psychiatrist can get involved in the commitment process is when dealing with a voluntarily hospitalized patient who wishes to leave the hospital, but who has shown ample evidence of meeting the criteria for commitment. The psychiatrist might then serve as a petitioner, or in some hospitals as both petitioner and examiner, in the commitment process. It should be clear from this brief description that psychiatrists who primarily see outpatients and psychiatrists employed by community mental health centers, as well as psychiatrists who deal primarily with inpatients, can become involved in the commitment process.

The material which the psychiatrist sends to the court must include statements as to why the psychiatrist believes the patient might be dangerous to himself or others and why he believes the patient is mentally ill or inebriate. As a general rule courts are more likely to recommend commitment if such reports are based on factual statements such as "the patient admits to having severely beaten his wife" or "the patient believes that all attorneys are CIA agents who are trying to kill him" than on the impressions of the psychiatrist. It is useful to make the report as thorough as possible. Like any psychiatric report that is designed to assist nonpsychiatrists, it should be as free of jargon as possible.

The psychiatrist's report will be used as evidence in some type of hearing. A few states now require that a probable cause hearing be held within a few days of the initiation of the commitment process. The main purpose of a probable cause hearing is to determine if there is substantial evidence that the patient meets the standards of involuntary hospitalization. If such evidence is found, the patient can be kept in the hospital until the major commitment proceeding is held. A final and the more procedurally complete hearing is usually held within ten to thirty days following the petitioning for commitment. At this hearing the court may decide that the patient can be restrained for a longer period of time, usually varying between thirty and ninety days. In most states the psychiatrist has the option of appearing at the hearings as a witness or merely sending his report. Appearing in court is an imposing drain on a psychiatrist's time. It is somewhat more likely, however, that the psychiatrist's recommendations will be followed if he is present in court.

With all the new protections of the patient's rights, the psychiatrist still retains considerable and relatively unmonitored power to restrain people for brief periods of time. Magistrates and clerks tend automatically to approve psychiatric recommendations to hospitalize until the issue of commitment is formally resolved. In states which provide for probable cause hearings, as much as two to seven days may elapse before they are conducted and the psychiatrist's recommendations are formally reviewed. In states which do not have probable cause or preliminary hearings, only a magistrate's approval is required to initiate the patient's hospitalization until a judicial hearing is held. In this situation the issue of the patient's committability may not be finally adjudicated for ten days or longer.

The psychiatrist also has the power to recommend release of a patient at any time during the commitment process. Whether serving as an examiner at a mental health center or psychiatric hospital, as an attending physician caring for a patient who is waiting for a commitment hearing, or as a physician tending to the needs of an already committed patient, the psychiatrist can discharge the patient whenever he believes the patient no longer meets the standards of committability and is ready to leave the hospital.

To summarize, the psychiatrist still retains power to restrain the patient for brief periods of time and to release the patient at any time. Only the courts, however, can sanction the confinement of patients for longer time spans, usually periods of over two weeks. When the question of whether or not·the patient is actually to be committed is being determined, the psychiatrist's role changes. He then becomes an expert witness or a person who simply conveys information to the court. He has no direct influence over the court's decision.

This system is characterized by some obvious inconsistencies. The standards for commitment in most states now require findings of both dangerousness and mental illness. A number of attorneys have argued (and have been supported in court opinions) that psychiatrists should have only a limited role in determining whether patients are dangerous, and that dangerousness should be decided entirely in the courtroom.[13] Yet the statutes of all states allow the psychiatrist to restrain people solely on his own judgment of the patient's dangerousness for at least forty-eight hours or longer. The legal authorities seem to be saying that the psychiatrist's judgment of dangerousness is adequate in the short run but inadequate in the long run. Or the courts may be recognizing that it is almost impossible to hold emergency hearings in the middle of the night or at any time immediately following the petition for commitment, and that the psychiatrist's judgment as to the need for hospitalization may be worth honoring for reasons of convenience.

There is also inconsistency in limiting the psychiatrist's power to influence the final decision for commitment, but at the same time giving psychiatrists almost total power to release the patient at any time. If it is assumed that psychiatrists are not knowledgeable enough to judge when a patient is dangerous and sick enough to be restrained, then it is difficult to argue that they do know enough to judge when illness and dangerousness have sufficiently receded so that the patient can be released. The inconsistency here may be related to our society's intense concern with the patient's liberties. The message seems to be that the courts are not as concerned with harm resulting to patients and others from releasing patients too soon as they are concerned with possible harm to a patient who is restrained unnecessarily. An eminent forensic psychiatrist, Dr. Robert Sadoff, has suggested that if the court assumes ultimate control of the commitment decision, the court should logically assume total responsibility for releasing the patient. Dr. Sadoff notes that this would at least protect the psychiatrist from the risk of malpractice should he prematurely release patients who harm themselves or others.[14] Although Dr. Sadoff is quite correct in pointing out the inconsistency of

---

[13]"Suggested Statute on Civil Commitment."

[14]R. Sadoff, "New Malpractice Concerns for the Psychiatrist," *Legal Aspects of Medical Care* 6, no. 3 (1968): 31–35.

current approaches, it is extremely unlikely that the courts would ever assume the cumbersome and expensive burden of making release decisions for all patients.

A final possible explanation of the inconsistencies in current commitment proceedings is that the courts, although espousing the necessity of the dangerousness standard, are still influenced by a belief in the older standard of the presence of mental illness and the need for its treatment. When the court allows a psychiatrist to have so much power in restraining a patient for several days with only perfunctory monitoring of that action, there seems to be a strong assumption that the psychiatrist has some expertise in dealing with acutely disturbed people and that the assumption of this role is justifiable in emergency situations. Similarly, when the courts allow psychiatrists to release committed patients without any monitoring whatsoever (other than the threat of malpractice litigation), they may be reflecting that lingering belief that psychiatrists do know something about mental illness and its treatment and can be trusted to decide which patients have been successfully treated.

What Are Some of the Theoretical Considerations Involved in the Shift Toward "Dangerousness" as a Criterion for Civil Commitment?

I have already noted that one major factor in the shift toward a "dangerousness' standard was the argument that the courts needed an "objective" standard for commitment and could not rely on the "subjective" reports of psychiatrists. But the impetus toward "objectivity" was created by a deep concern for the value of freedom.

In one of the most important decisions regarding civil commitment a federal court stated, "The power of the state to deprive a person of the fundamental liberty to go unimpeded about his or her affairs must rest on a consideration that society has a compelling interest in such deprivation."[15] There are two major arguments for society's having a compelling interest in depriving people of liberty. First, under the so-called *parens patriae* doctrine the state has traditionally assumed the power of guardianship over disabled persons. Under English common law this power initially was restricted to control of the property of mentally disabled individuals. From the middle of the nineteenth century until just recently the practice in the United States has been to expand the *parens patriae* doctrine so that the mentally ill could be restrained and treated in their own best interests. Self-destructive patients, gravely disabled patients unable to care for themselves, and patients assumed to lack com-

---

[15]Lessard v. Schmidt, 349 F. Supp. 1078 (E. D. Wis. 1972).

petence to make effective treatment decisions were usually committed under the *parens patriae* doctrine.

A second justification for depriving people of liberty is the necessity of protecting society from antisocial acts. The police power of the state can be invoked either to arrest and try antisocial individuals as criminals or to restrain people who are "potentially dangerous" and are likely to harm others because they are mentally ill.

Both the *parens patriae* and police power justifications of civil commitment have been thoroughly questioned by the courts.[16] A number of federal and state courts have questioned the competency of psychiatrists or anyone else to determine what is best for a patient and to invoke commitment in the patient's best interests. Except in instances in which recent suicidal behavior suggests that continued self-destructiveness is imminent (that is, the patient is dangerous to himself), the *parens patriae* doctrine is being increasingly rejected as a criterion for civil commitment. It is exactly around this issue, of course, that most psychiatrists would profoundly disagree with the reform-minded courts. Most psychiatrists are convinced that there are people who because of mental illness are unable to judge what is best for them. We assume that a humane society would wish to intervene and take care of these people. The federal courts have thus far taken a stand that the potential damage resulting from depriving such individuals of their liberty exceeds the possible benefits of their treatment.

As the courts increasingly reject the *parens patriae* doctrine, they are somewhat more comfortable in embracing the police power of the state as a justification for civil commitment. When we commit people to protect society, however, we must determine that they represent a threat to society. They must be "dangerous to others." There has long been a pervasive belief in our society that the mentally ill are more dangerous than others and that mental illness somehow or other causes dangerous behavior. This belief seems to have sustained the reform-minded courts' belief in the constitutional validity of restraining patients under the police power of the state.

Invoking the police power as a justification for commitment raises major problems. When we commit a person under police power justification, we are actually responding to his behavior as though he were a criminal. If we deprive him of freedom, it is primarily for our benefit, not his, and under our constitution that person should be entitled to the same rights as an offender facing a criminal sentence. Once we move from a *parens patriae* to a police power justification of civil commitment,

---

[16]*Ibid.*; Humphrey v. Cady, 405 U.S. 504, 509 (1972); Hawks v. Lazaro, 202 S.E.2d 109 (W.Va. 1974).

therefore, there is no alternative but to turn the commitment process into something resembling a criminal proceeding. And this, of course, is what has happened in recent years. *Parens patriae* justifications are still invoked in the commitment of those who are imminently self-destructive and less and less frequently in the commitment of those who cannot care for themselves. (The commitment of suicidal patients can in theory be partially justified by the police power of the state since suicide is a crime.) Psychiatrists, of course, still try to justify their involvement in the commitment process of nonsuicidal patients as largely serving a protective or *parens patriae* function. But this does not reflect the prevailing view of the courts that only dangerousness to self or others justifies commitment.

There are other constitutional problems involved in committing people under a police power justification. Such commitments involve detention of people who may not have committed a criminal act but who are only suspected of having that potentiality.[17] Preventive detention is considered an improper exercise of police power in this country. Society as a rule is reluctant to confine persons solely because of what they might do in the future. In no area other than that involving treatment of mental patients do we take such a cavalier attitude with regard to restraining people who have not committed a crime. The police power rationale for detention of people who have not committed crimes may eventually be seriously questioned as unconstitutional, particularly as it becomes increasingly clear that many of these people cannot be successfully treated in mental hospitals.

How Is Dangerousness Defined in Most Commitment Laws?

It is somewhat ironic that the switch to a dangerousness standard of commitment was partially justified by the argument that we needed more objective standards than the presence of mental illness or the need for treatment. In practice, "dangerousness" proves to be a more elusive concept than mental illness. Court decisions and statutes which include "dangerousness" as a standard do not provide careful definitions of the term. One immediate question with regard to defining dangerous behavior is whether it should be restricted to acts which result only in harm to other people or if it should include acts that result in harm to property. Another question which arises if dangerousness involves harm to people is whether there should be evidence of direct physical harm or if psychic harm to others should be included in the definitions.

[17]"Suggested Statute on Civil Commitment."

Once dangerousness is defined there is still the problem of how it will be detected. Courts and statutes have presented a variety of interpretations as to how dangerousness is determined. The trend is to view people as dangerous enough to be committed only where there is documented history of an overt act of "dangerous behavior" such as violence to others or a threat of violence. In dealing with dangerousness to oneself, the trend is to institute commitment only if there is documented evidence that the individual has already tried to harm himself or has threatened to do so. If there must have been an overtly dangerous act or threat before commitment can be instituted, there must be some guidelines which define for what limit of time such acts or threats can be viewed as relevant or useful predictors of the patient's future dangerousness. Obviously, if many weeks or months have elapsed since the occurrence of the dangerous/overt event, the risk of the patient's continuing to be dangerous may have long since passed. A relatively precise concept of dangerousness would provide guidelines which would help the courts determine for what period of time an individual is dangerous. Many of our current statutes tend to bypass this issue by providing for the commitment of the "imminently dangerous." Imminence is of course not definable, and even the model commitment statute of the American Bar Association does not speak of a definitive time period, but talks about the probability that dangerous acts will occur within the "near future."

Finally, no courts have ruled nor have any statutes specified what probability of harm must exist before a patient can be committed. The model commitment statute as prepared by the American Bar Association suggests that commitment is justifiable if it is more likely than not that in the near future the person will harm himself or others.[18] The "more likely than not" phrase suggests that there must be a greater than 50% probability that the person will hurt himself or others. As will be noted shortly, there is absolutely no means of making a prediction of harm to self or others with 50% accuracy.

Thus, dangerousness turns out to be a disturbingly imprecise standard. Criminologists who have studied the concept of dangerousness for decades have despaired of defining it, and some have warned that our preoccupation with the concept may stifle research and lead to repressive social actions.[19] In many jurisdictions dangerousness can now be about anything a particular court wants it to be. Undoubtedly much litigation and legislation in the next decades will be focused on experimentation with new views of dangerousness. It should be clear,

---

[18]*Ibid.*, p. 100.
[19]Y. F. Rennie, *The Search for Criminal Man* (Lexington, Mass.: D. C. Heath, 1978).

however, that the concept is so inherently laden with value judgments that any definition which is given legal sanction will be quite arbitrary.

Is Dangerousness Predictable, and Are Psychiatrists Any More Equipped to Predict It Than Anyone Else?

We do not know the extent to which dangerous behavior (assuming it has been defined) is predictable, and we do not know if psychiatrists have any special skills in predicting it. Research in this area is obviously limited by the legal and moral problems involved in doing predictive studies. Predictions that a given individual is dangerous usually result in his commitment or treatment. It is unlikely that society would ever condone allowing a matched control group predicted to have dangerous tendencies to be left alone untreated. If the committed or treated person then fails to commit a dangerous act, we do not know if the original prediction was wrong or if society's intervention diminished his dangerousness.

Given the problems with research in this area there have still been a number of follow-up-type studies done which define certain limitations and abilities psychiatrists bring to the predictive process. Our current knowledge can be summarized as follows:

1. There is an enormous legal and moral pressure on psychiatrists to overpredict dangerousness. Underprediction of dangerousness can result in tragedy. The safest course for the psychiatrist who wishes to spare his patients and others unnecessary death and suffering, and who wishes to avoid lawsuits, is to overpredict dangerousness.[20] Psychiatrists, like any group, tend to opt for the safest course.

2. There have been follow-up studies of individuals confined in institutions for large amounts of time because of suspected dangerousness who were later released by court order. Most of these individuals were not violent when released. These studies demonstrate rather convincingly that psychiatrists have little skill in predicting whether people who have spent a great deal of time in institutions will be violent once they have left the institution.[21]

[20]J. Monahan, "The Prediction of Violence, in *Violence and Criminal Justice*, edited by D. Chappel and J. Monahon (Lexington, Mass.: D. C. Heath, 1975).

[21]H. J. Steadman, "Employing Psychiatric Predictions of Dangerous Behavior: Policy v. Fact," in *Dangerous Behavior: A Problem in Law and Mental Health*, edited by C. J. Frederick (Rockville, Md.: NIMH, 1978).

3. The person who has a previous history of violent behavior is more likely to commit a violent act than the person who does not have such a history.[22]
4. One observer has suggested that the psychiatric predictions of dangerousness in the emergency room might have more accuracy than other predictions since the environmental variables involved in the ultimate occurrence of a violent act are more readily observable in that situation.[23]
5. Psychiatrists can predict that certain individuals are more likely than others to behave in a violent or self-destructive manner. In dealing with people who later harm others we cannot say with any certainty what this likelihood is. When it comes to predicting suicide we have a little more knowledge. It is likely that people who have made previous attempts at suicide are about one hundred fifty times more likely to kill themselves than people who have not. A person who is psychologically depressed is fifty times more likely to kill himself than the average person.[24]

The "state of the art" of predicting dangerousness can be summarized as follows. Certain people can be identified as being more likely than others to commit acts labeled as dangerous. And there are variables about which psychiatrists have some knowledge such as the patient's history, his mental status, and his habits, that help in this process of identification. We can provide the court with at least a little bit of data which may help them in their decision regarding commitment.

What psychiatrists must acknowledge is that we cannot predict violence very accurately in individual cases. Even when we can say that a person is fifty times more likely to commit suicide than the average person, that person is still unlikely to kill himself. If we predicted suicide in the case of every individual who showed high susceptibility, we would be wrong far more often than we would be right. In dealing with dangerousness to others our tendency to overpredict is likely to result in an even higher incidence of false positives than when we predict suicide.

As long as commitment decisions are framed in terms of the

---

[22]H. L. Kozol, R. J. Boucher, and R. F. Garofalo, "The Diagnosis and Treatment of Dangerousness," *Crime and Delinquency 18* (1972): 371–92.

[23]J. Monahan, "Prediction Research and the Emergency Commitments of Dangerous Mentally Ill Persons: A Reconsideration," *American Journal of Psychiatry 135*, no. 2 (1978): 198–202.

[24]A. Pokorny, "Suicide Rates in Various Psychiatric Diagnosis," *Journal of Nervous and Mental Disease 139* (1964): 495–505.

dangerousness standard, society must face the recurrent and agonizing question, "How many people do we want to restrain unnecessarily in order to prevent just a few from hurting themselves or others?" This is a political and moral question. Decisions as to how many people we want to deprive of freedom to save a few lives, or conversely, how many people we are willing to let die to preserve freedom, are truly awesome. Psychiatrists cannot and should not make such decisions. The use of the dangerousness standard should sharpen the psychiatrist's awareness that commitment is a legal and not a medical process.

Ideally psychiatrists should strive to conduct research which will enable us to expand the accuracy of statements we make to the court with regard to alleged dangerousness. As long as psychiatrists are required by law to make such statements in the course of their involvement in the commitment process, it is useful to seek ways of improving their accuracy. Someday we may be able to provide the courts with a relatively accurate probability statement of a given individual's likelihood of committing a dangerous act. (Sociologists can now make such probability statements with regard to the likelihood of criminal offenders' committing a subsequent crime. The probability is expressed in terms of percentages.[25] It is extremely unlikely, however, that our probability statements will ever reach a 50% level, and any court which expects an accurate prediction that a person is more likely than not to commit a dangerous act is relying on nonexistent expertise. (The psychiatrist's lack of expertise in this area is usually acknowledged by civil liberties attorneys.[26] Yet these same attorneys have helped to institute the dangerousness standard. Psychiatrists sometimes feel doubly oppressed by being forced to testify to a standard they have not created and then being criticized for not being able to do so with accuracy.)

In practice psychiatrists who participate in commitment proceedings should learn to be extremely modest in making statements about a patient's dangerousness. The experienced psychiatrist will acknowledge that there is no certainty that a prediction of dangerousness will be accurate and there is a considerable likelihood that it will be wrong. Whenever the law allows, the psychiatrist should focus on describing why he believes that a particular patient is more likely than the average person to commit a dangerous act and should avoid outright prediction of dangerousness.

[25]S. Shah, "Dangerousness and Mental Illness: Some Conception, Prediction and Policy Dilemmas," in *Dangerous Behavior: A Problem in Law and Mental Health*, edited by C. J. Frederick (Rockville, Md.: NIMH, 1978).

[26]Shah, "Dangerousness and Mental Illness: Some Conception, Prediction and Policy Dilemmas."

What Are Some of the Major Problems Created by the Dangerousness Standard?

There are six major problems involved in patient care and decision-making which are directly related to the emergence of the dangerousness standard. The first and certainly the most serious is that there are now many patients who are severely mentally ill, who suffer greatly, who are unable to make competent decisions to accept treatment, and who are definitely treatable, but who nevertheless are deprived of the opportunity of receiving treatment if they cannot be found to be dangerous to themselves or others. Patients with manic-depressive disorders fit into this category. These patients are frequently unwilling to be treated and yet they are very sick and quite treatable. Watching such a patient suffer, humiliate himself, squander his wealth, alienate his loved ones, or drastically compromise his future while resisting a treatment that would be of enormous help is an incredibly frustrating and heart-breaking experience for anyone who cares about people.

Other patients with severe but treatable psychoses, or with severe depression, are also denied access to treatment. The criterion of "imminent dangerousness" often makes it impossible to commit and treat people who are at high risk of suicide over a prolonged period. "Atrocity stories " involving this issue are plentiful. Depressed patients who deny suicidal intentions in court are almost always released before an adequate course of treatment can be completed. It is not uncommon for these people to kill themselves a few weeks or a few months after discharge by the courts.

A second problem with the dangerousness criterion is that it can encourage hospitalization of individuals who are not treatable. State hospitals are becoming populated with extremely violent patients who may have mild to severe mental illnesses for whom modern-day psychiatry has little effective treatment. In past years these individuals were sent to prison. Today the law makes it easier for them to be sent to a mental hospital. It is questionable whether these people are any better off in a mental hospital than in a prison. Certainly many mental hospitals are ill-equipped to care for them.

These patients are a serious management problem within mental hospitals. Sometimes they pose a physical threat to other patients and to staff. They certainly make the daily life of nondangerous patients unpleasant and unsafe. Patients committed as potentially dangerous often take up a great deal of the time of treatment staff. They are likely to be individuals who have major personality disorders and who are quite demanding of treatment resources even if they have been unresponsive to treatment. Dealing with such patients leaves doctors and other therapists with less time to work with those who are treatable.

A third problem with dangerousness criteria is that except in instances where the patient is clearly suicidal the psychiatrist has no useful guidelines to help decide who is committable. As noted previously the term "dangerousness" is usually defined loosely enough so that the psychiatrist has much discretion in initiating the commitment process. The discretion available to the psychiatrist is in many ways similar to that available to a policeman on a beat. Just as the policeman can make unmonitored decisions to arrest or not to arrest, the psychiatrist must make similarly decisions as to whether to initiate commitment or not to initiate commitment. But the policeman at least has certain clear standards in the form of laws to follow in making his decision. At one time the psychiatrist could rely on standards which directed him to act in the best interests of his patients. Today, however, the standards are nebulous. Many psychiatrists who work in the commitment process for a period of time make compromises with the judicial system or learn to manipulate it. Some psychiatrists learn to gauge their recommendations to the predilections of the particular judge who sees most of their patients. Others learn to initiate commitments which have little chance of being sustained just so they can get the patient hospitalized for a few days of treatment. Still other psychiatrists automatically initiate commitment of any equivocal case so that the court will have to assume responsibility for what is done to the patient. (Psychiatrists fear that if they release a patient who harms himself or others, they may be sued. They know that the judge cannot be sued.) Although psychiatrists have found ways of adapting to the new commitment standards, many of our adaptations put us in a manipulative role and are certainly not in the best tradition of medicine.[27]

A fourth problem is that adherence to the dangerousness standard gives certain types of exploitive patients considerable control of entry to and exit from the hospital. Patients who for a variety of reasons prefer temporary life in an institution to life in the free world now have an easy means of achieving quick entry. A patient need only threaten suicide to be admitted to a hospital. That same patient can usually gain quick release by simply stating that his suicidal proclivities have passed. Thus patients who for various reasons are having difficulties in surviving in the community because of difficulties with the law, coping with poverty, or wanting to escape a life situation they view as oppressive, tend to seek civil commitment. These patients can often be helped in a hospital setting, but they could also probably be helped by a more efficient sys-

[27]Ennis and Emery, *Rights of Mental Patients,* p. 47.

tem of social welfare or outpatient treatment. In past years, when commitment was primarily based on severe mental illness, psychiatrists did not worry too much about the threat of malpractice when they simply denied these patients admission. Today it takes an extremely courageous psychiatrist to deny admission to a patient who is making threats, even when the psychiatrist doubts that the threats are sincere.

A fifth problem with the dangerousness criterion is that it insidiously pushes the psychiatrist into an adversarial role with the patient. This is especially true when the psychiatrist must deal with patients who are alleged to be dangerous to others. In the process of initiating commitment of people who are dangerous to others the psychiatrist is largely serving society. He may be serving the patient at the same time, but his allegiances to society and to the patient are obviously divided. Psychiatrists have of course frequently found themselves in "double-agent roles," but usually this happens in situations where such roles can be clearly explained to patients and where the psychiatrist has the opportunity of placing his primary initiative on helping the patient.[28] If dangerous but treatable patients are committed, the psychiatrist can focus on treatment and remains, in part, the patient's "friend." The psychiatrist who participates in commitment of a nontreatable patient, however, can certainly be viewed as the patient's adversary. Even if the patient's condition should change so that he later became treatable he might be extremely reluctant to accept help from a professional he has viewed as a prosecutor.

A sixth problem is created by the manner in which the looseness of the definition of dangerousness leads to disparate practices on the part of psychiatrists which may eventually harm patients. Some state hospitals, understaffed and not wanting to be troubled with difficult patients, have simply taken to developing extremely rigid definitions of dangerousness and are unlikely to retain anyone in the hospital unless there is considerable evidence that he is going to hurt himself or others within the next few hours or days. (There is a small risk of malpractice in such situations, but as noted previously, the hospital psychiatrist can release a patient at any time and the courts exercise no restraint on this power.) At the same time, psychiatrists in private practice or in academic settings may develop more liberal definitions of dangerousness which conflict with those of state hospital psychiatrists. They may initiate commitment of patients who are quickly released by the state hospital. The patient is then shuttled about needlessly because of a conflict between doctors. It should not be surprising to find psychiatrists fighting with one another

[28]S. L. Halleck, *Psychiatry and the Dilemmas of Crime* (New York: Harper and Row, 1967).

over this issue. When treatment facilities are understaffed, the interests of the doctor who has to care for the patient may be quite different from the interests of the doctor in the clinic or in private practice who initiates commitment. The dangerousness criterion is sufficiently vague as to leave much room for argument between members of our own profession in situations where we have some discretion to retain or release the patient. It is doubtful that such disagreement helps patients.

Finally, it is conceivable that the dangerousness criterion may play an insidious role in sustaining a racist approach to patients. Alan Stone has noted that nonwhites are not nearly as overrepresented in state hospitals as they are in prisons.[29] Apparently factors related to race have in the past made it more likely that deviant nonwhites would go to the prison rather than the hospital. It is likely that the dangerousness criterion will perpetuate this inequity.

Black members of my hospital staff have recently called to my attention the infrequency with which blacks are committed as dangerous to others. A number of these patients have subsequently committed crimes and been sent to prison. Apparently some courts view the violence of blacks as being "normal" or syntonic with their culture as long as the violence is directed toward other blacks. (This is not a new phenomenon. The criminal courts have long been known to be liberal in dealing with violence of blacks as long as it was directed toward other blacks.) These same courts are frequently willing to commit white patients whose violent propensities seem to be minimal.

In Actual Practice Are There Ways of Getting around the Dangerousness Criterion and Initiating Commitment on the Basis of the Patient's Needs and Treatability?

In the ACLU handbook *The Rights of Mental Patients*, Bruce Ennis states, "Because statutory definitions of dangerousness are usually vague, it is easy for mental health professionals to call people dangerous. As we noted, many professionals consider dangerousness a mere technicality, a magic word that must be uttered in order to 'get patients the treatment they need.' Psychiatrists often lable prospective patients 'dangerous' in order to achieve parens patriae purposes."[30]

Mr. Ennis is correct. Some psychiatrists have undoubtedly used the vague wording of dangerousness standards to "fudge" and try to obtain treatment for people who are not dangerous but who might be benefited by treatment. The psychiatrist can do this with a relatively clear con-

[29]Stone, *Mental Health and Law.*
[30]Ennis and Emery, *Rights of Mental Patients,* p. 47.

science when definitions of dangerousness are sufficiently vague. Often the psychiatrist may not even be aware of "fudging," and may unconsciously exaggerate or expand the concept of dangerousness.

It is regrettable that psychiatrists have to resort to imaginative definitions of dangerousness in order to achieve humanistic purposes. It is also unwise and ultimately unproductive to do so. The courts in most jurisdictions will eventually settle on their own definitions of what they consider to be dangerous behavior. Over a period of time the opinions of psychiatrists whose definitions of dangerousness differ from those of the courts will routinely come to be rejected.

What Issues Are Involved in Responding to the Mental Illness Standard in Civil Commitment?

While all states continue to require a finding of mental illness as a condition of involuntary commitment, the statutory definitions of mental illness offered as guidelines are vague. This should not be too surprising because there is much disagreement among psychiatris⁺ʒ in defining mental illness. Up until now I have argued that the concept of dangerousness is more nebulous than the concept of mental illness, but this does not mean that precise definitions of mental illness are readily available. It is relatively easy for a psychiatrist to find some justification for placing almost any person in one of the categories listed in *DSM II*. If the psychiatrist utilizes the newer *DSM III*, the range of behaviors listed as mental disorders is even greater (a person who abuses tobacco or who occasionally has insomnia can be classified as mentally ill under the proposed draft of *DSM III*).[31] It is especially easy to fit people who are suspected of being dangerous to self or others into some kind of diagnostic category. People who have made suicide attempts or threaten suicide are likely to be depressed and are easily defined as having affective disorders or character disorders. People who harm others or threaten to harm others are relatively easily defined as having impulse control disorders or personality disorders. It takes just a little creativity on the part of the psychiatrist to find some diagnostic classification for the allegedly dangerous patient. And it is also unusual for the courts to question the psychiatrist's findings of mental illness too rigorously.

A number of mental health attorneys have provided guidelines for attorneys who wish to discredit psychiatric testimony regarding diagnosis.[32] While these make interesting reading, they are rarely utilized in

[31]Task Force on Nomenclature and Statistics, American Psychiatric Association, "DSM III—Draft" (Washington, D.C.: APA, 1978).
[32]J. Ziskin, *Coping with Psychiatric and Psychological Testimony* (New York: Law and Psychology Press, 1975).

practice. As a general rule the psychiatrist's statements regarding mental illness go unchallenged, and judicial disagreements with psychiatrists are confined to the area of dangerousness. The dangerousness issue in general dominates the commitment proceedings and distracts the court from looking at the severity of the patient's illness or the extent of his suffering.

It is my belief that if dangerousness were not a criterion for involuntary commitment there would be more pressure on psychiatrists to provide rigorous evidence for the existence of mental illness and the need for the patient to receive care or treatment. I also believe that psychiatrists could meet this challenge. Competent and reliable diagnosis of mental illness would, however, require that psychiatrists define only the most severe emotional disorders as mental illnesses. Civil liberties attorneys are fond of arguing that psychiatrists disagree about diagnoses and that there is little reliability in the entire field of psychiatric diagnosis.[33] They tend to quote studies which support this thesis and to ignore studies which refute it. Actually, the reliability of diagnosis in psychiatry is comparable to its reliability in other medical specialities as long as the studies are restricted to the more severe emotional disorders, namely, organic brain disease, functional psychosis, or severe depression.[34] As a general rule it is the above categories of the most incapacitating emotional disorders which are most likely to compromise the patient's competency to make rational decisions regarding treatment—and which are most likely to be treatable.

In summary, the mental illness criterion of commitment is currently vague enough so that it can be used to justify the commitment of many who might not need treatment and who might not benefit from it. When combined with the criterion of dangerousness the mental illness standard is especially prone to be used sloppily. Restricting involuntary commitment to patients who have only severe and treatable emotional disorders would eliminate these problems.

How Is It Possible to Commit Patients Who Are "Gravely Disabled"?

Some states still allow for the involuntarily commitment of patients who in addition to being mentally ill are unable to care for their physical needs. Such "gravely disabled" patients, unable to find ways of meeting

[33]D. D. James, "Handling the Civil Commitment Case," *Mental Disability Law Reporter 2*, no. 4 (1978): 456.
[34]J. Helzer *et al.*, "Reliability of Psychiatric Diagnosis: A Methodological Review," *Archives of General Psychiatry 34* (1977): 129–33.

basic needs for food and shelter, are viewed as dangerous to themselves. Grave disability is most likely to be seen in elderly patients with organic brain syndromes who resist the efforts of others to help them. Even the most staunch civil libertarians tend to tend to agree that under the *parens patriae* doctrine the state has some obligation to care for these people. There is disagreement, however, as to whether "grave disability" should be a standard for involuntary commitment or whether such disability should be handled by having the patient declared incompetent and by appointing a guardian to care for him.[35]

In most states people who are unable to care for themselves can be declared incompetent. A guardian or conservator is then appointed who must arrange for services to meet the patient's needs. While the guardian will explore all possible ways of helping the patient function outside of an institution, sometimes the guardian must recommend hospitalization. In such instances hospitalization, even though imposed on the patient, is viewed as "voluntary." The guardianship provision offers an interesting alternative to involuntary commitment for providing services to those who may be incompetent. It is often an acceptable alternative to civil liberties attorneys even though the reasoning involved in the guardianship process is reminiscent of that involved in the now unpopular *parens patriae* doctrine of civil commitment. (Apparently attorneys are more troubled by the state's assuming power to treat involuntarily. In the guardianship procedure that power is, at least technically, assumed by a caring person, not the state.) The legal issues involved in the use of guardianships will be discussed in a later section.

Is There Legal Justification for Involuntary Commitment of Patients Who Are Primarily Nuisances to Others?

As of this writing only a few states expressly provide for commitment on the grounds of protecting the "welfare" of others. Protection of the public welfare leads to control of offensive or unpopular people. Our society is too often intolerant of certain variations in lifestyle. We sometimes define practices which are annoying to the majority of people as evidences of illness and then commit people who engage in such practices on the grounds of protecting the welfare of others. Commitment of young people who are involved in lifestyles offensive to their more conservative parents would be one example. Such commitments certainly have political meaning, but they can also be viewed as efforts

---

[35]"Legal Issues in State Mental Health Care: Proposals for Change," *Mental Disability Law Reporter* 2, no. 1 (1977): 88.

temporarily to rid society of "nuisances." There is never any moral, medical, or legal justification for commiting a patient whose behavior is merely offensive to others unless the patient is also mentally ill, treatable, and incompetent. It is quite likely that all states will soon change their laws to provide for commitment criteria which are too rigorous to allow for commitment of nuisance patients. While the criteria legislated may not be desirable, all professionals should welcome the disappearance of frivolous commitment.

How Well Do Current Standards of Commitment Serve to Protect Political Activists from Involuntary Commitment for Political Reasons?

There has been much concern in recent years over the practice of confining political prisoners to mental hospitals rather than prisons. This practice is common in the Soviet Union, and some fear that the commitment process can be abused in the same manner in this country.[36] Defining a dissenter as a sick person rather than as a person who breaks the law in order to further a cause tends to negate the power of that person's dissent. It is also conceivable that in a mental hospital (as contrasted with a prison where an offender is sent for a fixed period of time) the political dissident might be restrained indefinitely.

With the new procedural safeguards (to be discussed in the next chapter) now available to those facing involuntary commitment, it would seem unlikely that political dissidents in America could be shunted to mental hospitals rather than be allowed to remain free or go to prison. It should be noted, however, that the new standards for civil commitment do not in themselves provide protection for the political dissident. Political activists make statements and promote acts which can easily be construed as dangerous to others. I have noted previously that the courts, when faced with the dual criteria of mental illness and dangerousness, tend to focus primarily on dangerous behavior and do not demand rigorous definitions of mental illness. Political dissidents might be safer from hospitalization under a legal system which demanded more rigorous proof of severe mental illness. As things stand now, political dissenters who commit illegal acts can too easily be defined as mentally ill, and their main safeguard from a politically repressive commitment is their procedural rights.

[36]T. Szasz, *The Manufacture of Madness* (New York: Harper, 1970).

8

The Rights of the Mentally Disabled

The recent change in the standards for involuntary commitment represents only one of the many changes designed to protect the rights of the mentally disabled. These days the patient is provided with many of the same procedural rights in the course of the commitment process that the accused offender receives in the course of a criminal trial. A person charged with a crime is granted certain protections during the procedures which determine his guilt or innocence. He is entitled to make maximum use of these protections to ensure that he will not be punished unless it can be proven that he is guilty. In the civil commitment process procedural rights are designed to ensure that people who do not meet the standards for commitment will not be involuntarily hospitalized. Some of the rights now granted patients have little influence on the practice of psychiatry. Psychiatrists as a rule do not oppose these rights, and usually favor them. Some of the new rights, however, generate consequences which should concern us. Conducting the civil commitment process in the same manner as a criminal proceeding can produce a variety of situations and outcomes which are definitely not good for patients.

Civil liberties attorneys like to argue that the new reform movement in mental health law is simply an extension of the humanistic concern for the rights of offenders which arose in the 1950s and 1960s. The attorneys seek to "rescue" their clients from the mental health system with the same (and sometimes even more) determination attorneys evidence in their efforts to protect criminal clients. It is sometimes difficult to know why they are so enthusiastic and why there has been so little questioning of the use of the criminal justice model in making decisions to treat the mentally ill. Alan Stone has noted that the system now proposed as a model for dealing with the mentally ill has hardly been effective in dealing with criminals.[1] Our system of criminal justice is notoriously ineffective in controlling crime, and neither does it regularly dispense justice to all classes of people in a fair manner. More important, the system survives only by virtue of its capacity to divert the majority of its subjects from the actual trial process. If we are to adopt the criminal justice model in dealing with the mentally ill it is important to know how the former system is sustained through the process of diversion.

Actually only a tiny percentage of those indicted for committing a felony end up having a trial. The great majority of cases are either dismissed or "plea bargained."[2] If efforts were made to have a full adversarial hearing for every person arrested and charged with committing a felony, our states and municipalities would be faced with a completely unmanageable financial burden. Once a person is convicted of a crime the criminal justice system can also divert him from institutional care by such devices as probation, suspended sentences, or work release. If this form of diversion were not available, our expenditures for prisons would be staggering.

To the extent that the mental health system becomes modeled after the criminal justice system, expenses quickly get out of hand unless the new procedural rights are in large part ignored (thereby saving court costs) or more patients are diverted from the system. Any legal system which relies on adversarial procedures must eventually "streamline" its procedures or develop a means of getting rid of an overflow of cases. These is no analogy to plea bargaining in civil commitment cases. Diversion from the mental health system can only be accomplished by discouraging the initiation of commitment proceedings. There are still a few jurisdictions in which the new procedural rights may be provided in only a perfunctory way, but for the most part the courts have dealt with the overflow problem in the mental health system by discouraging commitment. This would not be objectionable if community services were available which could effectively treat the patient who is not committed. However, many patients who need hospitalization cannot be treated in the community, and community resources are usually lacking for those who could benefit from outpatient treatment.

Finally, it is discouraging to note how those who embrace the criminal justice system as a model for dealing with the mentally ill have failed to note basic differences in the purposes of dealing with criminals and the mentally ill. The criminal law is designed to impose retribution or

[1]A. Stone, "Recent Mental Health Litigation: A Critical Perspective," *American Journal of Psychiatry 134*, no. 3, (1977): 273–79.
[2]R. H. Kuh, "Balancing the Scale of Justice: How to Make Plea Bargaining Work," *The New Leader*, January 1974.

punishment on the offender, to deter him and others who might be tempted to commit similar crimes, to incapacitate him temporarily in order to protect society, and to rehabilitate him. The first two purposes, retribution and deterrence, require that substantial penalties be imposed on anyone found guilty. Society has a clear wish or need to inflict a certain amount of psychological pain upon the criminal. Since punishment is an inevitable part of the criminal justice process, it is absolutely essential that those who are truly innocent be protected from the risk of being found guilty. But the mental health system is not set up to serve functions of retribution or deterrence. It exists primarily to rehabilitate those who are disabled, and sometimes to incapacitate temporarily those who might harm themselves or others. Certainly the patient may experience the consequences of involuntary commitment as aversive, and sometimes they are, but this is an unfortunate and usually temporary outcome of the process rather than a goal. Indeed, the goals of the criminal justice system and the mental health system are usually antagonistic. The former seeks to inflict psychological pain upon its clients and the latter seeks to diminish their mental anguish. Given these realities, the patient should not logically require the same degree of legal protection from the aversive consequences of involuntary confinement as the accused offender. This is not simply a theoretical argument. Involuntary patients live in far more comfortable environments than prisoners. They have better food, better housing, better recreational facilities, and better medical care. Most important these days, they have far greater physical safety. Rape, assault, extortion, and murder rarely occur in hospitals but are endemic to our prisons. Those mental health lawyers who talk about involuntary hospitalization's imposing as much or more suffering upon people as imprisonment have simply never spent much time observing conditions in prisons or hospitals.

What Implications Does Providing Patients Facing Commitment with the Right to Counsel Have for Psychiatric Practice?

Most states now provide patients facing involuntary hospitalization with a right to counsel, and many states require that a lawyer be appointed to assist the patient who contests hospitalization. For the most part this is a desirable and rational change. The patient who is represented by an attorney has a certain degree of protection in the commitment process. Attorneys can often prevent unnecessary hospitalization by questioning inaccurate assessments of the patient's condition, and can sometimes assist the patient in finding ways to solve his problems in extrahospital settings. The mere fact that a patient has an attorney at a commitment hearing substantially lessens the probability that the patient will be committed.[3] To the extent that attorneys help prevent unnecessary commitments and help provide patients with alternative solutions to problems, their involvement in the commitment proceeding is fortunate for all concerned. The patient's right to counsel, however, has also created some problems. One problem is cost. The services of attorneys do not come cheaply and the expansion of due process in the commitment process has created an expensive new industry. Another problem is that attorneys have difficulty deciding whether to serve the best interests of their patient or simply to do what their clients request. When the patient is incompetent his best interests may be poorly served by following his requests. Until recently many attorneys faced with a completely irrational and incompetent patient were willing to assume a guardianship role and to assist in the process of helping the patient obtain treatment with the least possible restriction of freedom. In recent years, however, several courts have ruled that attorneys representing patients should serve solely as their advocate.[4] This means that the attorney is legally required to follow the wishes of people who may be severely mentally incapacitated and in fact incompetent to make decisions regarding treatment. The move toward requiring attorneys to adopt an unyielding advocacy role is based on the erroneous assumption that all people at all times are competent and can make self-serving decisions. It puts attorneys in the unfortunate position where they must argue for judicial outcomes which are clearly damaging to their clients. Not surprisingly, younger attorneys who are most likely to do the daily work involved in representing patients are beginning to question the morality of their roles.[5]

What Relationship Should the Psychiatrist Who Is Treating a Patient Have with an Attorney Who Is Representing the Patient?

There are no clear answers to this question. As a rule the patient's attorney will not try to contact the psychiatrist, but the two parties may encounter one another on a hospital unit before the hearing takes place. Some psychiatrists will refuse to have anything to do with the patient's attorney. Even though the attorney is entitled to visit with the patient

[3]T. J. Scheff, *Being Mentally Ill* (Chicago: Aldine, 1966).
[4]"Guidelines for Defense Counsel in Commitment Cases," *Mental Disability Law Reporter* 2, no. 4 (1978): 427–30.
[5]L. P. Galie, "An Essay on the Civil Commitment Lawyer: Or How I Learned to Hate the Adversary System," *Journal of Psychiatry and Law*, Spring 1978, pp. 71–87.

and review the patient's records, he cannot insist on discussing the case with the psychiatrist. Other psychiatrists are quite willing to talk to the patient's attorney and often entertain a hope that they can influence him to cooperate in ascertaining that the patient receive proper treatment. This approach is not entirely naïve. Many attorneys are deeply moved by the emotional plight of their clients. A few have a certain amount of sophistication with regard to mental illness and all are troubled by the thought that they might do something to hurt their clients. On the basis of information received from psychiatrists, attorneys sometimes try to persuade their clients to accept hospitalization and treatment. It is also possible, however, that the attorney may use the interview with the psychiatrist solely to pick up any clues that might be viewed as evidence against commitment and totally ignore the medical and humanistic arguments advanced by the psychiatrist.

My own practice is to talk with the client's attorney when I have the time and to present him with as objective a picture of the patient's condition as I can. I have few illusions that I am going to convince many attorneys to function as guardians rather than as advocates, but I do feel that it is important that the attorney receive a clear message as to the potential harm he may inflict upon the patient by pursuing the advocacy role too vigorously. At least part of my intention here is educational. I want the attorney to know something about the depths of suffering involved in mental illness and I want him to feel some responsiblity for the adverse consequences of his advocacy position.

Should the Psychiatrist Who Is Involved in the Commitment Process Have His Own Counsel?

Even with all the recent changes, procedures in the commitment process are still not identical to criminal justice proceedings. One critical difference is that the commitment process, although now more adversarial, is still a process in which only one side has legal representation.[6] In most jurisdictions there is no attorney representing the state's interests. Efforts are certainly made to put the psychiatrist in the prosecutorial role and sometimes psychiatrists have unwittingly accepted that role. This is unfortunate.

I firmly believe that the psychiatrist should never accept a role as adversary to the patient. Acceptance of such a role is a denial of the reality that the psychiatrist's decisions must always be partially or totally

[6]Commission on the Mentally Disabled, American Bar Association "Suggested Statute on Civil Commitment," *Mental Disability Law Reporter* 2, no. 1 (1977): 143.

based on his perceptions of the patient's best interests. Psychiatrists who participate in the commitment process do, of course, contribute to a social control function. But from the psychiatrist's perspective the controls imposed on a patient are necessary only insofar as they facilitate treatment. Stated differently, the psychiatrist's only legitimate role in the commitment process derives from a *parens patriae* rather than a police power theory of involuntary hospitalization. (Conceivably, under current laws a psychiatrist may cooperate in the commitment process of dangerous patients for whom he believes no help is available. I would urge psychiatrists to reject this role whenever possible.) None of this should be taken to mean that patients will not at times experience the psychiatrist primarily as someone who deprives them of freedom. The problem here is that patients perceive only one facet of the psychiatrist's role and are unwilling or unable to appreciate other aspects of that role. The patient's experience of the psychiatrist as totally adversarial represents a distortion which should not be reinforced by law.

It is likely that in the near future more states will appoint attorneys to represent the state's interest in the commitment process. This may bring a certain equity to the adversarial process in commitment hearings. It may also take a certain amount of pressure off psychiatrists who now get pushed into a prosecutorial role. The psychiatrist, however, should strive to avoid viewing the state's attorney as his representative. *In legal proceedings, the psychiatrist should always view himself as a rather humble servant whose role is simply to present the court with rational suggestions for being helpful to the patient. Beyond his compassionate interest in the welfare of the patient, the psychiatrist should have no personal interest in the outcome of the commitment hearing. From the psychiatrist's standpoint nobody but the patient wins or loses a commitment hearing.*

What Effects Does the Patient's Right to a Judicial Hearing Have on Psychiatric Practice?

Aside from the possibility that hearings will sometimes require psychiatrists to spend a great deal of time in court and away from patients, the right to a judicial hearing has little direct influence on psychiatric practice. It is a right which patients obviously need. The possibility that psychiatrists may spend more and more time in court and have little time to treat patients is, however, serious. Although most states still do not require the psychiatrist's actual presence at the hearing and are willing to accept his written report, it is unlikely that the courts in their expanding commitment to the use of the criminal justice model will continue to allow psychiatrists such luxury. It should be noted that recent trends would lead to the psychiatrist's being involved in two types of hearings: the probable cause or preliminary hearing, which would take place shortly after the patient's hospitalization; and the final hearing, which would be a much more formal proceeding taking place sometimes ten days to a month after admission.

How Does Giving the Patient Notice with Regard to Hearings Influence Psychiatric Practice?

The current trend is to allow patients at least one day's notice prior to a probable cause hearing and several days' notice prior to a final hearing. The person facing commitment is entitled to a written notice in language he understands which states the time and place of the hearing, the name, address, and telephone number of the attorney who will represent him, the statutory standard on which he may be committed, the rights he has prior to a hearing and at the hearing, the reasons and the specific facts that are alleged to justify commitment, the names of all persons who will testify in favor of hospitalization, and the substance of their testimony. While all this is certainly time-consuming, it should have no negative effects on the mental health of patients and no important influence on psychiatric practice. Most psychiatrists would probably agree that giving patients notice as to judicial hearings is simply a humane, logical, and probably therapeutic responsibility of the mental health system.

What Are the Implications for Psychiatric Practice of Allowing Patients to Employ Their Own Expert Psychiatric Witness at a Commitment Hearing?

If civil commitment is to be an adversarial process, and if psychiatrists are to testify as experts that a patient should be committed, it seems reasonable that psychiatrists might also testify as experts that the patient should not be committed. To the extent that psychiatrists are asked to testify as to the issue of dangerousness they are likely to disagree with one another. This should not be surprising. We know so little about dangerousness that psychiatrists, like any other group of professionals or nonprofessionals, will interject their own political and moral biases into their assessments and will come up with differing predictions. To the extent that experts disagree as to the prediction of the

dangerousness of a given individual the commitment process may become more complex and interesting. It is unlikely, however, that a battle
of experts over an issue where there is no expertise is likely to be of
much help to the court or to the patient.

On the other hand if psychiatrists were to focus their testimony on
the issue of the severity of the patient's mental illness, its treatability,
and its prognosis, different psychiatrists might through their examinations of the patient come up with different kinds of data. There might
be disagreement here, but it would be disagreement over issues which
can be studied scientifically. If the patient employs a psychiatrist who
happens to disagree over diagnostic issues with the psychiatrist who
recommends commitment, neither should feel too uncomfortable about
airing their differences. It is always possible that the psychiatrist recommending commitment has made a diagnostic error. The patient is
simply given the opportunity to have a second diagnostic opinion and
the court may gain information which will be useful in making its decision.

If the criminal justice model continues to prevail in the civil commitment process, more psychiatrists may wish to serve as expert witnesses for patients contesting commitment. There is nothing wrong with
this as long as the psychiatrist hired by the patient, just like the psychiatrist who initiates commitment, clarifies his limitations of expertise regarding dangerousness and tries to confine his expert testimony to areas
involving mental illness, a subject about which he should be knowledgeable.

Do Patients Have a Right Not to Be Medicated before Their Judicial Hearings?

There is a widespread belief among civil liberties attorneys that
patients who receive medications before their hearings are somehow or
other less able to present a good appearance before the court and assist
their counsel.[7] These attorneys paint a picture of the medicated patient
as a "zombielike" creature who is likely to come across to others as
mentally ill simply as a result of having taken medication. Certainly an
overmedicated patient can sometimes look strange and unattractive, and
may have difficulty in thinking clearly. If patients are adequately diagnosed, however, and medications are used according to reasonable med-

[7]B. J. Ennis and R. D. Embry, *The Rights of Mental Patients* (New York: Avon Books, 1978),
p. 73.

ical standards, it is likely that the mentally ill patient who is receiving medication will be in a better position to plead his case than the patient who is not. Often the highly disturbed patient can present a rational appearance in court only if he is properly medicated. Unfortunately, it is not unheard of for a psychiatrist on occasion to welcome the opportunity to accede to the patient's request to go to court without medication in the hopes that the patient will be more likely to show his "craziness" and be committed. While commitments sustained on this basis may be helpful to patients in the long run, doctors should not be proud of participating in a process in which the condition of patients is deliberately allowed to deteriorate.

In this day and age it is likely that most severely disturbed individuals will need treatment with medication as soon as there is reasonable certainty about the diagnosis. There is something inherently inhumane about keeping these people locked up for as long as ten to thirty days without medication because of a belief that this will help them at a hearing. The right to refuse medication before a hearing can lead to needless suffering on the part of severely disturbed patients and may even compromise their chances of avoiding commitment. It is worth noting that this particular right might become superfluous if the courts continue to legitimate the right to refuse treatment. If the courts rule that any patient not adjudicated incompetent can refuse any form of treatment, the patient facing commitment will usually be able to refuse medication.

Does the Patient's Right to Be Present at a Judicial Hearing Have Any Implications for Psychiatric Practice?

The only reason that might justify keeping a patient out of a hearing is a high probability that the hearing would so upset the patient as to worsen his condition significantly or perhaps elicit disruptive behavior in the courtroom. It is usually difficult to predict how a patient will respond to the stresses of a courtroom appearance. Patients who are disturbed in the hospital may behave more normally in court and patients who behave normally in a hospital may behave quite irrationally in court. In the absence of accurate predictability in this area, the most rational approach would be to welcome the current right of patients to be present at their own hearing if they so wish. The risk of the patient's being psychologically traumatized at a judicial hearing can be lessened by placing the patient on appropriate medication (as long as the law still allows doctors to do this).

How Might the Emerging Demands That Patients Have the Right to Be Protected against Self-Incrimination in the Commitment Process Influence Psychiatric Practice?

While the courts have thus far not moved to protect patients from facilitating the process of their own commitment, arguments for providing patients with the right against self-incrimination under the Fifth and Fourteenth Amendments are becoming more strident[8] Here again the issue is whether the commitment of a psychiatric patient is analogous to the conviction of a criminal. If it is assumed that the processes are similar or identical, the patient as well as the offender must be protected from self-incrimination. The psychiatrist who examines the patient and makes a recommendation for commitment can then be viewed as taking a role similar to that of a police officer interrogating a suspect. Once the psychiatrist is viewed in this way, it follows that the patient would be entitled to three types of protection. First, he would need to be warned that whatever material he revealed to the psychiatrist could later be used to document the case for his eventual involuntary commitment. Second, he would need the right to have an attorney present at the time of the psychiatric examination. And third, he would need the right to remain silent during the examination if he felt he could incriminate himself or if he were advised to remain silent by his attorney.[9]

If privileges against self-incrimination ever become a reality, it might be necessary for psychiatrists to give all patients a *Miranda*-type warning prior to the beginning of an interview as to the possible consequences of the doctor's recommendations. This would not be a major problem when the psychiatrist is functioning as an examiner in the commitment process. It is often good clinical practice to allow competent patients to know what consequences can arise from interviews conducted by psychiatrists who are in a double-agent role. Of course the situation is different in an emergency room or outpatient situation where the psychiatrist may end up being the petitioner and is likely to hear the information which leads him to initiate commitment in an unexpected and inadvertent manner. It would be absurd for the psychiatrist to warn every patient he sees in every conceivable setting that material revealed during every psychiatric examination or interview might result in the patient's commitment.

Hopefully, even if patients are eventually provided with a right against self-incrimination it will only apply to the psychiatrist who

[8]"Suggested Statute on Civil Commitment," pp. 101–05; F. W. Miller *et al., The Mental Health Process* (Mineola, N.Y.: Foundation Press, 1976), pp. 379–82.
[9]Ennis and Embry, *Rights of Mental Patients,* pp. 74–76.

functions as an examiner who is an agent of the state or the court. Most agency-employed psychiatrists would have no difficulty in adhering to this requirement if they were given some discretion to waive the warning in dealing with incompetent or highly disturbed patients. (The examiner could make his decision to waive the warning on the basis of information provided in the petition and others' observations of the patient.) It has been my experience that competent patients appreciate the doctor's honesty in this situation and that full disclosure as to the potential uses of the doctor's report does not discourage communication. In fact, it may increase the patient's trust in the doctor and his willingness to reveal problems. [10]

The presence of an attorney during a psychiatric interview might bother some psychiatrists but would not trouble others. Many of us are used to interviewing in front of groups, and as long as the attorney remains silent and merely takes notes he would not interfere with the diagnostic process. In my own work I would welcome the presence of attorneys when I examine with regard to possible commitment. If the patient is severely disturbed, the sensitive attorney might perceive the patient's need for treatment and might be persuaded to act in the patient's best interests.

If the patient has a right to remain silent during a psychiatric interview, is advised to do so by his attorney, and follows this advice, the consequences for the patient could be much more grim. It is not possible adequately to evaluate a noncommunicative patient. Providing the patient with a right to remain silent could result in the exclusion of medical input from the entire process of commitment and treatment.

The critical issue in this whole area is whether the psychiatric examination is more similar to a police interrogation designed to incriminate the patient or to a diagnostic process designed to help the patient. In terms of goals and methods it would be absurd to consider it anything but the latter. Certainly in the emergency room or clinic the psychiatrist does not even think about commitment until an evaluation has been made. The psychiatrist is first of all trying to decide what is wrong with the patient. Second, he thinks about treatment. If he decides hospitalization is necessary to meet treatment goals, he assumes that in the majority of instances the patient will accept voluntary treatment. There is usually no dealing with the possibility of initiating involuntary commitment until the examination has ended, treatment has been suggested, and the patient has rejected it. Only at this point will the psychiatrist begin to ask the patient questions which may be relevant to the issue of involuntary treatment. Like the petitioning psychiatrist, the court-

---

[10]S. L. Halleck, *Psychiatry and the Dilemmas of Crime* (New York: Harper, 1967).

appointed psychiatrist who examines the patient after the petition has been made must be much more concerned with diagnosis and treatment than with issues relating to the patient's need for confinement. His first obligation is to find out what is wrong with the patient and how the patient can best be treated. No rational decision with regard to commitment can be made until this is done. The assumption on the part of some attorneys that the psychiatrist uses an examination to incriminate a patient is based on a view of the psychiatrist as a person who is concerned only with society's needs and not with the patient's needs. This view represents a gross distortion of reality.

Of all the rights that have been granted or are being requested for patients, the right of patients to remain silent to prevent self-incrimination is potentially the most harmful to their well-being. The examination of the patient often provides evidence of the existence of treatable illnesses. Often, the existence of these illnesses cannot be suspected, investigated, or confirmed unless the patient is able to communicate with the doctor. Thus, patients who follow their attorney's advice not to cooperate in the psychiatric examination risk their health and their lives. The most frightening scenario one can visualize if a right against self-incrimination is sustained is that of a patient with a potentially fatal illness, such as a subdural hematoma or encephalitis, who develops symptoms which bring him to a psychiatrist and then is told by an attorney not to cooperate in the diagnostic examination. In such a situation the presence of the acute brain syndrome which might quickly have been suspected by virtue of the patient's performance in the psychiatric interview would very likely be missed in an ordinary physical examination. In advising such a patient not to communicate with the physician in fulfilling his advocacy function, an attorney would be assisting the patient to an early death.

How Would Imposing Rules of Evidence Requiring Limitation of Hearsay Testimony Influence Psychiatric Participation in the Commitment Process?

Hearsay evidence is information which is not based on personal knowledge of the witness but is a repetition of what the witness has heard others say. Its value is dependent not only on the veracity of the witness but on the veracity and competency of other persons as well. Psychiatric reports and medical reports are based rather heavily on what family members, nurses, nursing assistants, social workers, and psychologists say about the patient. In legal terms, a certain proportion of the content of any psychiatric report would be considered hearsay.

As a rule, hearsay evidence is not allowed in a criminal proceeding.

Secondhand evidence is not valued as highly as original evidence, and the person who originally produced the evidence cannot be present for cross-examination. If the physician's report is viewed as an adversarial document which in effect indicts the patient, it obviously should not be allowed to include hearsay statements. On the other hand, if it is viewed an ordinary medical report, the material it includes which was not obtained firsthand can simply be considered as extremely useful information which facilitates decision-making as to the patient's diagnosis and treatment.

With the new interest in applying criminal procedures to the commitment process there is an increasing demand on the part of civil liberties attorneys to exclude hearsay material from psychiatric reports and have the doctor testify only as to what he has actually observed personally. Such a doctrine, if implemented, might require the courtroom appearance of nursing personnel, social workers, and psychologists who have observed various forms of maladaptive behavior and whose observations are usually incorporated in the doctor's reports. Those who favor the use of the criminal process in dealing with mental patients face a severe dilemma here. Adherence to criminal court procedures would require subpoenaing a large number of witnesses who are actively involved in patient care. This would maximally protect the patient's rights, but would also massively expand the legal process at the expense of treatment. Some civil liberties attorneys have suggested that the problem could be resolved by holding commitment hearings at hospitals so that all staff involved in treating the patient could be subpoenaed without having to travel to court.[11] Even such a compromise, however, would still require a great deal of diversion of professional treatment time to the courtroom. A procedural right might, again, be damaging to the patient.

Would Providing the Patient Facing Commitment with a Right to Trial by Jury Substantially Influence Psychiatric Practice?

The right to a jury trial is now available by statute to patients facing commitment in some states. Some federal courts have also recently heard appeals for providing the patient with the option of a jury trial. It is hard to see how this particular right could have a major influence on psychiatric practice. The only important issue here is time. The jury trial could take more time than a trial heard only by a judge, and the right to a jury trial could make new demands on professional time.

[11]"Suggested Statute on Civil Commitment," p. 107.

Are Changes in the Standards of Proof in the Commitment Procedure Likely to Influence Psychiatric Practice?

In civil cases the standard of proof is the "preponderance of evidence." In tort law, for example, if the fact finder believes it is more probable than not that a given individual is negligent, then that individual is liable. In criminal cases, where the issue of an individual's liberty is critical, the more stringent standard of "beyond a reasonable doubt" is applied. The "beyond a reasonable doubt" standard permits some defendants who are actually guilty to go free so that few defendants who are actually innocent will go to prison. Society would rather suffer the consequences of criminals' walking the streets than increase the chance that liberty will be unjustly compromised.

Again it is the switch to criminal justice standards in the civil commitment process that has led to demands for higher standards of proof. In a recent case before the United States Supreme Court it was argued that commitment must be supported by proof of a need for confinement "beyond a reasonable doubt" rather than by "a preponderance of the evidence."[12] The court compromised on this issue and required an intermediary standard of "clear, cogent and convincing" proof, but state courts are still allowed to insist on the higher standard of "beyond a reasonable doubt."

The demand for legislating higher standards of proof seems to be just one more absurdity which arises when the commitment process is "criminalized." The "beyond a reasonable doubt" standard of proof might sometimes be met if the question at issue was "Is this patient mentally ill?" But as long as the courts commit according to a standard of dangerousness, it would seem unlikely that the psychiatrist or anyone else could provide evidence beyond a reasonable doubt that a patient is dangerous. If proof "beyond a reasonable doubt" is demanded, it would seem that only those who have just committed a crime or self-destructive act and are threatening to repeat it could logically be committed.

What Is the Doctrine of Least Restrictive Alternative as Applied to Psychiatric Patients, and How Does It Influence Psychiatric Practice?

The Supreme Court has ruled that the state cannot impose any greater restrictions on fundamental freedoms than are necessary to serve

[12]Addington v. Texas, U.S. 77-5992 (1979).

a legitimate state interest or purpose.[13] As applied to civil commitment this principle has been translated into the doctrine that the state must use a setting for treatment which entails the least restriction necessary on the patient's freedom.[14]

In effect, the least restrictive alternative principle requires that involuntary control of patients involve no greater restriction on freedom of movement than is necessary for treatment and protective purposes. If an individual can be more effectively treated in a halfway house, in a group home, or by remaining with his family, he should be allowed to remain in this less restrictive setting. Some federal courts have ordered state hospitals and state mental hygiene systems to develop alternative and less restrictive means of treatment.[15] This usually means community or outpatient treatment. The courts have also argued that the patient must be treated with the "least drastic means" available.[16] This aspect of the least restrictive doctrine has been used to justify the case for the regulation of certain forms of treatment and for the patient's right to refuse treatment.

At first glance it might seem that psychiatrists would want to embrace the least restrictive alternative doctrine. Good practitioners are aware of the patient's need for freedom and try to use the most benign treatment. The major problem here, however, is that the least restrictive treatment is not always the most effective treatment. Some patients could probably be treated in halfway houses but not nearly as humanely or efficiently as in hospitals. Depressed patients might eventually recover with psychotherapy but they are more likely to recover quickly with somatic treatments. In its most literal and absurd form, the doctrine of least restrictive treatment puts a well-intentioned but irrational restraint upon medical practice. It ignores parameters such as compassion and efficiency. It may be good law, but it can lead to bad medical treatment.

The "least restrictive" doctrine has had some interesting implications for the development of community resources. In many communities patients in need of treatment could be taken care of in nonhospital settings if there were adequate community resources. But often such resources are not available. A number of suits have been initiated based on the least restrictive alternative doctrine which have called for improved community resources.[17] Some civil liberties attorneys have

[13]Shelton v. Tucker, 364 U.S. 479, 488 (1960).
[14]D. Chambers, "Alternatives to Civil Commitment of the Mentally Ill: Practical Guidelines and Constitutional Imperatives," *Michigan Law Review 70* (1972): 1107.
[15]Stone, "Recent Mental Health Litigation."
[16]Wyatt v. Stickney, 334 F. Supp. 1341, 1343–44 (M.D. Ala., 1971).
[17]Dixon v. Weinberger, 405 F. Supp. 974 (D.D.C. 1975).

argued that if the community is unwilling to provide less restrictive alternatives, patients should simply not be committed. This argument can, of course, become just one more legal ploy for keeping all types of people out of the hospital. On the other hand some reform-minded lawyers have joined psychiatrists in arguing that the least restrictive alternative doctrine imposes a legal obligation on the community to create better care facilities.[18] In a few instances mental health professionals have worked together with reformers of the mental health bar to secure judicial orders that pressure state legislators and city councils to appropriate funds to provide a full array of community-based alternatives.[19] Their efforts have thus far had minimal success.

What Are Some of the Legal Issues Psychiatrists Must Consider When Dealing with Voluntary Hospital Patients?

The majority of psychiatric patients enter the hospital willingly and their treatment is rarely complicated by the kind of legal involvements associated with the treatment of involuntary patients. Of course, few patients enter the hospital with great enthusiasm. Most patients come because they are too frightened to try to deal with their problems outside the hospital or because they are simply taking their doctor's advice. Civil liberties attorneys sometimes refer to these patients as nonprotesting patients rather than as voluntary patients.[20] This term has the invidious and inaccurate connotation that all such patients are hospitalized under duress.

Some patients classified as voluntary, however, do have little choice as to whether they enter or remain in the hospital. Some patients enter psychiatric hospitals to avoid the consequences of criminal actions. Children, as will be noted later, can be committed as "voluntary" patients by their parents. Incompetent individuals can be committed as "voluntary" patients by their guardians. And, of course, a certain number of patients sign into a hospital "voluntarily" because they know that if they do not, commitment proceedings will be initiated against them. It is this latter group in particular whose voluntariness must be questioned and whose rights and possible loss of rights most concern the civil liberties reform movement.

[18]R. J. Bonnie, "Commentary: Criminal Responsibility," in *Diagnosis and Debate,* edited by R. J. Bonnie. (New York: Insight Communications, 1977), p. 295.
[19]A. Stone, "The Right to Treatment and the Psychiatric Establishment," *Psychiatric Annals* 4, no. 9 (1974): 43–50.
[20]B. J. Ennis, "Legal Rights of the Voluntary Patient," *Journal of the National Association of Private Psychiatric Hospitals,* Summer 1976.

Voluntary mental patients are treated differently from physically ill patients. The mental patient cannot simply leave the hospital whenever he wishes. As a rule he signs a form when he comes into the hospital wherein he agrees that he can be restrained for a certain period of time after he requests to leave. Even the patient who willingly admits himself to the hospital can be required to remain anywhere from forty-eight hours to thirty days after the time he requests a discharge. The limitation on the voluntary patient's freedom to leave the hospital at any time can sometimes be helpful in the patient's treatment. A patient who enters the hospital voluntarily may shortly after admission experience a deterioration in his mental condition, become frightened, and want to leave the hospital. Often the patient wants to leave at exactly the time when he is in most need of treatment. The forty–eight–hour to thirty–day restraining period (thirty days, incidentally, is extraordinarily lengthy; I cannot think of a way to justify a restraining period of over seventy-two hours) does give the doctor a chance to observe the patient, to try to persuade the patient to stay in the hospital, and to initiate commitment proceedings if these turn out to be absolutely necessary.

The major problem here is that patients who enter the hospital voluntarily often do not know that they cannot leave at any time. There is a serious informed consent issue here. No patient should ever be allowed to enter a psychiatric hospital without knowing exactly what he has to do to leave and what restrictions might be placed on his departure. There is a tendency for doctors to be somewhat sloppy about providing this kind of information, and civil liberties attorneys are quite correct in deploring the voluntary hospitalization of competent patients which is not based on full informed consent.

What Is the Right to Treatment Doctrine as Applied to Psychiatric Patients?

The "right to treatment" doctrine was first advanced by Dr. Morton Birnbaum in 1960.[21] He argued that if the state involuntarily confines someone under the benevolent theory of *parens patriae,* then it ought to provide treatment. Dr. Birnbaum was seeking to bring the standard of treatment in public mental hospitals up to that available in private institutions. He tried to develop constitutional arguments for his basically moral position, but had little success. The first major case in which the right to treatment was upheld was argued in the District of Columbia in

[21]M. Birnbaum, "The Right to Treatment," *American Bar Association Journal* 45 (1960): 499–505.

1966. Judge Bazelon, a federal district court judge, relied on the statute under which the plaintiff, Rouse, was committed to argue for a statutory right to treatment.[22] In this case Judge Bazelon was merely trying to ascertain that a person being held in confinement for long periods of time receive some kind of effective therapeutic intervention. He noted the possibility that there might be a constitutional basis for the plaintiff's receiving treatment, but went no further in his opinion.

The first major case involving a constitutional argument for a right to treatment was tried in 1972.[23] In *Wyatt* v. *Stickney*, a class action suit was filed against the state of Alabama for provision of more adequate treatment to all patients confined to what was at that time a disgracefully understaffed hospital. This suit was the first right to treatment suit filed by an ordinary mental patient rather than one commited under a sex crime statute or a criminal insanity statute. It was heavily supported by a number of mental health and civil liberties organizations, and it was based on constitutional arguments. As a class action suit it involved all the patients in the hospital and raised the possibility that the state of Alabama would have to spend a great deal of money. The court in *Wyatt* essentially held that civilly committed persons in Alabama had a constitutional right to receive treatment or to be released from confinement. It ordered the implementation of a detailed series of medical and institutional standards designed to require state institutions to provide what was called a constitutionally adequate level of treatment. Since the *Wyatt* decision in 1971, several similar cases have been argued in other states where entire mental health systems have been required to expand services to the involuntarily confined. Legal scholars are still arguing whether the right to treatment is in itself a constitutional right or if it is simply "triggered" by situations in which patients are deprived of liberty. The argument which currently seems most popular is that patients cannot be involuntarily deprived of liberty or put in any situation of jeopardy or harm without having certain protections in the form of decent treatment and decent standards of living.

The Supreme Court has not ruled on the question of a constitutional right to treatment, but in the now-famous case of *O'Connor* v. *Donaldson* the court declared that the state could not constitutionally confine a nondangerous mentally ill individual "without more" and one interpre-

[22]Rouse v. Cameron, 373 F.2d 451 (D.C. Cir. 1966).
[23]Wyatt v. Stickney, 325 F. Supp. 781 (M.D. Ala. 1971), 324 F. Supp. 1341 (1971), 344 F. Supp. 373, and 344 F. Supp. 385 (1972); *Wyatt, Appeal Docketed Sub. Nom.* Wyatt v. Aderholt, no. 72-2634 (5th Cir. Aug. 1, 1972) *was consolidated for purposes of appeal with* Burnham v. Department of Public Health 369 F. Supp. 1335 (N.D. Ga. 1972). *Decision rendered at* 503 F.2d 1305 (5th Cir. 1974).

tation of the word "more" in this context is the presence of adequate treatment.[24] The *Donaldson* case involved a malpractice suit against a psychiatrist under section 1983 of the U.S. Code, a civil rights statute. Here, damages were awarded to the plaintiff, Donaldson, because the defendant, O'Connor, had failed either to treat or to release the plaintiff although opportunities to do either had allegedly been sufficient. Whereas the *Donaldson* case provides some support for the right to treatment concept, it is different from the *Wyatt* case and other similar cases. In *Donaldson*, there was an actual lawsuit against a doctor primarily responsible for treatment. In all the other right to treatment cases, although doctors had been named as defendants, they were primarily functioning as state agents and the suits were primarily against the state. In the latter cases, no damages were asked but the plaintiff's agenda was to use court injunctions to induce the state service and its medical representatives to implement changes.

The current trend in right to treatment litigation is for the federal court to compel the state mental health system and the plaintiffs to negotiate and to draw up what are called consent decrees which are then signed by the judge.[25] These decrees are actually guidelines of the attorneys of the Mental Health Law Project who initially represented the plaintiff in *Wyatt*. To a large extent they were interested in improving the plight of the involuntarily hospitalized. They also, however, wanted to get committed patients out of hospitals. Some believed that the state of Alabama would be unwilling or unable to comply with the right to treatment obligations and that one way the state could deal with the suit would be simply to release involuntarily committed patients.

Professional groups have had varying interests in right to treatment litigation. Most mental health professions other than psychiatry have supported right to treatment suits. Usually they are simply seeking better treatment for patients (although it has been suggested that the department of psychology at the University of Alabama was instrumental in pressing the *Wyatt* case because it wished to maintain professional control over teaching programs at Alabama hospitals).[26] Psychiatrists have been "fence sitters" on this issue. One reason we have taken a rather ambivalent stance is that some right to treatment suits name psychiatrists as defendants (although these are not malpractice suits but

---

[24]O'Connor v. Donaldson, 422 U.S. 563, 95 S. Ct. 2486, 45 L.Ed. 2d 396 (1975).

[25]Harvard Law Review, "Mental Health Litigation: Implementing Institutional Reform," *Mental Disability Law Reporter 2*, Nos. 2–3 (1977): 221–33.

[26]S. Stickney, "Wyatt v. Stickney: The Right to Treatment," in *Diagnosis and Debate*, edited by R. J. Bonnie. (New York: Insight Communications, 1977), pp. 274–81.

are requests for injuctions or court orders in which the psychiatrist as administrator is simply asked to carry out a charge).

The states, not surprisingly, have taken a defensive posture toward right to treatment suits. Implementing right to treatment orders requires expenditures of large sums of money. State legislatures have argued that they should not be bound to spend their citizens' money as a federal court directs. Often the commissioner of mental health, who is likely to be a psychiatrist, is caught between the demands of the court and the resistance of the state government. This is not a pleasant position for any administrative psychiatrist and is at least one factor contributing to a rapid turnover of psychiatric administrators in state mental health systems.[27] It is also true that federal courts are not ideally equipped to implement the details of treatment programs. Sometimes the courts try to enforce standards which seem quite arbitrary to the institution-employed psychiatrist.

The right to treatment doctrine has had a major effect on health care in those states in which it has been litigated, and has also influenced health care in other states. Since the original "Wyatt decision many states have sought to remedy inadequacies in the provision of mental health services. While right to treatment litigation has undoubtedly imposed a tremendous burden on mental health administrators and has probably resulted in premature release of seriously disturbed patients, psychiatrists would do well to view such litigation as ultimately advantageous to patients and to support it in selected instances. It is not, after all, always bad for patients to be discharged to the community if they are being involuntarily hospitalized at institutions which provide no treatment anyway. Viewed in its best light, the right to treatment doctrine is simply a moral argument that mental hospitals should provide adequate treatment. While it is necessary to remain alert to the conflicting motivations of various participants in right to treatment cases, individual psychiatrists and organized psychiatry can contribute to the betterment of patient care by advocating right to treatment standards which are sound, reasonable, and capable of being implemented.

Some psychiatrists have worried that the right to treatment doctrine could spawn a series of lawsuits against psychiatrists who work in crowded state hospitals and who cannot adequately treat all of their patients. There is actually little danger that this might happen. Psychiatrists, like any state administrators, may be open to sanctions of the federal courts when they do not follow court orders. But so far no administrator has been punished. The courts realize that administrators are caught between their orders and the will of the legislatures, and have

[27]Stone, "Recent Mental Health Litigation," p. 276.

been patient. Lawsuits similar to *Donaldson* are also unlikely. The real error in this case was related more to unnecessary confinement than to lack of necessary treatment. With all the current legislation protecting patients it is unlikely that the courts will allow prolonged confinement without treatment (as, strangely enough, they did in *Donaldson*). Today the courts would be most likely to order release, and malpractice issues would never be raised.

Do Psychiatric Patients Have the Right to Refuse Treatment?

All nonpsychiatric patients who are competent have the right to refuse treatment. In nonpsychiatric medical practice the imposition of treatment on a nonconsenting competent patient is likely to lead to a malpractice suit in the form of battery. The practice in dealing with psychiatric patients has been somewhat different. Until recently it was not uncommon even for voluntary patients who had not been adjudicated incompetent to have treatment forced on them. It has long been customary practice to impose involuntary treatment on committed patients.

In the past decade some federal courts have ruled that even legally committed patients have a right to refuse certain forms of treatment.[28] The early rulings in this area established the right of criminally insane and committed offenders to be protected from highly intrusive and sometimes experimental procedures such as psychosurgery and aversive behavior therapy. More recent federal court rulings have also questioned the use of more conventional treatments as provided to ordinary civilly committed patients.[29] As of this writing it is not clear whether a committed patient can refuse a conventional treatment such as antipsychotic or antidepressant medication.*

Civil liberties attorneys have been extremely creative in developing a case for the unconstitutionality of forced treatment. They have pointed out that in some instances enforced treatment might violate the constitutional right to privacy. In other cases it has been argued that the First Amendment provides patients with the right not to have treatments applied to them which would interfere with their thought processes and

[28]Mackey v. Procunier, 477 F.2d 877 (9th Cir. 1973); Knecht v. Gilman, 488 F.2d 1136 (8th Cir. 1973).

[29]L. H. Roth, "Judicial Action Report," *Psychiatric News 14*, no. 9 (1979): 3; R. Plotkin, "Limiting the Therapeutic Orgy: Mental Patients' Right to Refuse Treatment," *Northwestern Law Review 72* (1977): 465–82.

*As this book was in press both a federal and state court ruled in favor of the plaintiff's right to refuse certain medication.

religious beliefs. Eighth Amendment arguments have been used to describe some forms of psychiatric treatment as cruel and unusual punishment, and the Fourteenth Amendment has been cited in a case in which a patient was not given adequate procedural protection prior to placement in a treatment program.

Some observers feel that in states where commitment statutes are written so that the approval of commitment implies a certain degree of incompetency on the patient's part, the hospital may have the power (or perhaps even the obligation) to provide treatment to the nonconsenting committed patient. It is not certain, however, that the doctor can go ahead and treat a nonconsenting patient even in these states. In most other states at this time the physician treats a nonconsenting patient (even though the patient is committed) at some risk of malpractice. There is still no problem in treating a committed patient with conventional treatments such as drug therapy when an emergency situation threatens the patient's life. In most jurisdictions there is also little problem in going ahead with treatment if the patient is abusive and violent on the hospital unit and is threatening the safety of himself and others. But until the law becomes clearer, each psychiatrist would be wise to check current practices in his own state and to be extremely conservative in imposing treatments on the nonconsenting patient. Certainly, right now there is considerable risk in treating a nonconsenting, committed patient who is not creating any difficulty on the ward.

The above relatively dispassionate description of the current situation regarding the right to refuse treatment does not convey the grim consequences which result from such rulings. Having patients forced into a hospital situation where treatment is available, but where treatment cannot be given, is certainly not good for patients and is highly destructive to the morale of hospital employees. Allan Stone has noted that the right to refuse treatment litigation threatens to return our hospitals to the barbaric situation they were in one hundred years ago.[30] A scenario in which doctors cannot treat patients and in which highly disturbed individuals simply exist on psychiatric units is already a reality in some hospitals.

The problem here again is related to the reliance on a criminal justice model and the standards for committment which it has created. If people are committed under the police power of the state because they are dangerous to others and mentally ill, it is possible that some of them might not be treatable. We should not impose treatment on these people when it is not designed to help them. The right to refuse treatment makes sense when people are not treatable. The commitment of non-

[30]Stone, "Recent Mental Health Litigation," p. 278.

treatable people could be avoided, however, by rejecting the police power doctrine and basing commitment only on a *parens patriae* doctrine. Under a *parens patriae* doctrine involuntary hospitalization would be viewed as only one aspect of a broad treatment process. The process of commitment would be viewed as one designed to provide all varieties of treatment and the patient who has been adjudicated to be in need of treatment would have no right to refuse it.

Does the Patient's Right to Refuse Treatment Vary with the Type of Treatment?

Certain treatments are viewed by the legal profession, the courts, and some state legislatures as more "intrusive," "hazardous," or "harsh" than others.[31] Currently, the use of psychosurgery, electroconvulsive therapy (ECT), or some forms of aversive behavior modification are rigidly controlled by statute in several states.[32] Some states specifically prohibit psychosurgery or ECT for people under a certain age whether they consent or not. (At one time the state of California even tried to put legal controls on the use of ECT for consenting adult patients.) Other states have rather complicated incompetency and guardianship proceedings which must be utilized before the nonconsenting patient can be treated with ECT. While there are no objective data available on this issue, most psychiatrists believe that these laws have led to considerable diminution in the usage of ECT. Paradoxically, the new legalism has seemed to have the most significant influence on the use of ECT with poor people. Hospitals which deal with relatively affluent patients are usually sufficiently well staffed so that their professionals can take the time to go through the often tedious procedures of declaring the patient incompetent and finding him a guardian. On the other hand, understaffed state hospitals are often unable to provide the manpower to go through the incompetency and guardianship procedures. As a result, ECT is being used much more frequently these days in private hospitals than in public institutions.

There is currently much hope on the part of reform-minded attorneys that right to refuse treatment rulings by the higher courts will lead to the passage of statutes which control drug therapy in much the same way as ECT is currently regulated. In Minnesota efforts have already

---

[31]"Regulation of Special Techniques That Warrant Strict Scrutiny in Involuntary Treatment," *Mental Disability Law Reporter* 2, no. 1 (1977): 122–26.

[32]A. Brooks, "Mental Health Law: The Right to Refuse Treatment," *Administration in Mental Health* 4, no. 2 (1977): 90–95.

been made to declare prolixin therapy an intrusive procedure.[33] The amount of legal regulation which will eventually come in this area is still uncertain.

Psychiatrists, of course, resent the regulation of interventions by legal judgments as to whether they are intrusive, hazardous, or harsh. Most of us feel that we can assess the risks and benefits of a given treatment without the assistance of attorneys. The courts truly lack expertise in determining what is the best treatment for a given individual. While there may be an excellent argument for requiring legal supervision of all involuntary treatment, control of specific treatments on legal rather than medical rationales has absurd consequences. Electroconvulsive therapy, for example, is often a far safer and more effective treatment than many forms of pharmacotherapy. Yet attorneys have unreflectively assumed that it is a highly dangerous procedure and have been influential in controlling its use. One way to illustrate attorneys' lack of sophistication about ECT is simply to quote what the official American Civil Liberties Union handbook on the rights of mental patients says about it. The book states: "The procedure is simple: powerful jolts of electric current are used to shock the brain. Unconsciousness and at least one violent convulsion follow. Afterward, memory of up to several weeks prior to the treatment is lost, sometimes forever. Occasionally, the convulsions cause broken bones, particularly when muscle relaxing medications are not administered. Usually, the long-lasting effects are not so profound as the effects of psychosurgery. But many patients view electric shock as torture."[34] The above statement, which any medical student would appreciate as being at least fifteen years out of date, was published as part of an official guide for attorneys and patients in the year 1978.

How Can Incompetency Proceedings Which Provide Legal Sanction for Treating Nonconsenting Patients Be Initiated?

The procedure varies from state to state. In some states incompetency is still viewed as a global concept, and in order to have a patient adjudicated incompetent to refuse treatment the patient must also be declared incompetent to do most other things including administering his own finances, voting, making a will, or even marrying. This is especially unfortunate in states where the patient's status as incompetent

---

[33]T. K. Zander, "Prolixin Decanoate: Big Brother by Injection," *Psychiatry and Law*, Spring 1977, pp. 55–74.

[34]Ennis and Embry, *Rights of Mental Patients*, p. 139.

may be sustained for long periods of time even though he makes a quick recovery. More enlightened states have moved toward creating laws which allow for functional definitions of incompetency. It is possible in these states to adjudicate the patient to be incompetent to make a decision as to whether to accept or refuse treatment. The patient can then be treated involuntarily but retain all other aspects of legal competency. The legal proceedings involved in determining incompetency are often complicated. Proceedings can be initiated either by the patient's relatives, the concerned parties, or by the physician. Often, the final adjudication of incompetency requires a jury trial and can be extremely time-consuming. Most states, however, also have a provision for emergency adjudication of incompetency which can be used in life-threatening situations.

Once the patient has been adjudicated incompetent, the court can appoint a guardian who in effect makes the treatment decision for the patient. Legally the patient no longer has the power to refuse treatment and the guardian provides the "voluntary" consent for the patient. Of course, in this situation the guardian must be given full knowledge of the risks and benefits of treatment so that his consent is truly informed.

By What Standards Does a Court Judge Competency to Refuse Treatment?

Even in states which have statutes that talk about specific or functional competency regarding issues such as acceptance or refusal of treatment, there are no clear standards for determining such competency. Psychiatrists can provide some data which will assist the courts in determining incompetency, but there is no way of knowing how such information will be used. As a general rule, patients who are unresponsive and do not indicate a choice as to whether they desire or do not desire a treatment tend to be viewed as incompetent.[35] Sometimes the courts use a "reasonable man" criterion and try to decide whether a reasonable person would want to have the kind of treatment that is being offered. At other times the courts will be concerned with the possibility that the patient has an irrational reason for refusing treatment, such as a specific delusion about the possible harmfulness of the treatment or a psychotic condition characterized by severe self-destructiveness. In still other instances the court seeks to assess the patient's ability to evaluate the risks and benefits of treatment.

[35]L. H. Roth, A. Meisel, and C. W. Lidz, "Tests of Competency to Consent to Treatment," *American Journal of Psychiatry* 134, no. 3 (1977): 279–84.

Psychiatrists can certainly assist the courts by providing whatever information is known as to how the patient's current mental condition differs from his premorbid state. These kinds of data would be of some value when the court is trying to decide if the patient is behaving reasonably in refusing treatment. A patient who has always been scrupulous in taking care of himself, who has always sought medical attention even for minor ailments, and who suddenly begins to stop caring for his health and to resist all suggestions of treatment without saying why, may be judged to be behaving unreasonably. Psychiatrists can also explain to courts how various distortions of reality may lead to an irrational refusal of therapy. Finally, psychiatrists can probably contribute a great deal in pointing out how various mental illnesses distort the patient's perception of the risks and benefits of a given treatment and make for an incompetent evaluation of risk–benefit ratios.

With the emergence of stringent regulations of commitment and with the new emphasis on the patient's right to refuse treatment, it is likely that determinations of the patient's competency will begin to take on increased importance in psychiatric practice. This is an area which is relatively uncharted. Psychiatrists, like attorneys, have been prone to think of incompetency in rather global terms and have not wrestled with the problem of developing criteria for determining specific types of incompetency such as incompetency to refuse treatment. In effect the incompetency doctrine properly administered can accomplish many of the *parens patriae* goals of civil commitment. This is one topic about which we can anticipate a greatly increased dialogue between the courts and the psychiatric profession.

What Legal Changes Are Currently Influencing Psychiatric Care of Children?

The rights of children who become involved with the mental health system have expanded markedly in recent years. In many ways the debate over the involuntary confinement and treatment of children mirrors the debate regarding adults. The question of an individual's competency to act in his own interests is at the core of both controversies. With children it is somewhat easier for our society to accept the argument that someone other than the patient may be most able to make decisions which further the patient's best interests. It is unlikely that even the most ardent civil libertarian would argue that a five- or six-year-old child can make competent decisions regarding his psychiatric treatment. The issue, of course, becomes more complex as the child grows older. It is especially difficult to determine who knows what is best for an adolescent.

In some circumstances adolescents are fully capable of behaving like autonomous adults. In other instances they actively need external control and develop indirect ways of finding it. It is something of a truism in our society that adolescents often make demands for autonomy and independance which are not commensurate with their needs and which may not even reflect their internal motivations. The adolescent who tests limits by making demands and who then feels a powerful sense of relief and reassurance when they are refused is familiar to every parent, educator, or psychiatrist. Excruciatingly difficult situations arise when this familiar behavior pattern is misunderstood and it is assumed that the child's verbalized requests are always based on self-interest. As will soon be noted, the new legal trend is to accept the verbalized statements of a child as a true expression of his actual needs and wishes. For many children this practice has devastating psychological consequences.

The expansion of the rights of children began with efforts to protect them from unjustified commitment to training schools. Many training schools are simply prisons for youthful offenders. Yet in most states a child can be sent to a training school until he reaches the age of majority. For young adolescents this can mean an indeterminate sentence lasting up to several years. Ambiguities as to whether commitment to a training school is treatment or punishment pervade the juvenile law. In many states children can still be committed to a training school for "waywardness," "incorrigibility," truancy, promiscuity, or running away from home. None of the above "conditions" or behaviors is actually a crime under the adult criminal code, but if children commit such offenses they are in jeopardy of commitment to what are basically correctional institutions. In 1967 the Supreme Court provided certain procedural rights to adolescents facing commitment to a training school.[36] These were the rights for notice, counsel, the privilege against self-incrimination, and the right of confrontation and cross-examination. In 1970 the Supreme Court ruled that standards of proof in decisions involving juveniles sent to training schools should be similar to those used in the adult criminal justice process, that is, the standard for commitment should be "beyond a reasonable doubt," not merely "a preponderance of the evidence."[37]

These changes have been welcomed by the helping professions, including psychiatry. Juvenile training schools as a rule provide little or no treatment. The rights of children were being drastically compromised by the assumption that their commitment to a training school was as much a form of treatment as punishment, where their need for treatment was not always apparent, and where actual treatment was practi-

[36]*In re* Gault, 387 U.S. 1 (1967).
[37]*In re* Winship, 397 U.S. 358 (1970).

cally nonexistent. (It is important to note that protecting children from unnecessary commitment to training schools is not like keeping children out of hospitals. It is unlikely that very many children are helped by being sent to a training school and there is little likelihood that the "wayward" child will be harmed by not being sent to a training school.)

Because the correctional practices imposed on children have usually been cloaked in a treatment model, the courts have often been uncertain as to when they should send a disturbed youth to a mental hospital instead of a training school. Mental health and correctional facilities for children seem on superficial examination to be somewhat alike. (In some states training schools for children have been regulated by the state department of mental hygiene rather than by the state department of correction.) In past years courts, under the assumption that the child would have the opportunity for treatment in either type of institution, were prone to use nonmedical and nonlegal criteria in recommending one type of institution or another. Too often they based their recommendations on sociological variables (such as socioeconomic class and race) rather than on the needs of the child. As the courts became more aware of the deficiencies of training schools and more concerned with the rights of children as well as adults, it was inevitable that they would begin to focus on the rights of children to resist any kind of institutionalization, including hospitalization.

Except under certain carefully defined circumstances (which have been delineated in the section on malpractice) a child cannot consent to treatment and cannot consent to hospitalization. If a child is to be hospitalized it must be with the consent of his parents or legal guardians, who in effect "volunteer" their child into the hospital. Even if the child is resistant to the procedure, he is still considered a "voluntary" patient. As of this writing it is still true that in most states parents may place their children in mental hospitals without any form of judicial proceeding.[38] The only monitoring of the parents' decision is left up to the admitting physician. Once hospitalized, the child has difficulty in being released without the consent of the parent.

There is always a possibility that harm can result to the child in such a loosely monitored system. A particularly troubling concern is that an adolescent might be hospitalized by parents who wish to control that child's offensive or nuisance-type behavior by defining the child's deviation from parental norms as a form of illness. There is also some danger that hospital psychiatrists do not provide a sufficient check against such inappropriate admissions. If the psychiatrist becomes too identified with

[38]"Mental Health Treatment for Minors," *Mental Disability Law Reporter 2*, no. 4 (1978): 461.

the needs of the parents rather than those of the child, he may not be objective in evaluating the case for hospitalization. While there has been considerable exaggeration of the possibility that psychiatrists will be insensitive to the parents' use of an illness model to deal with an unruly child, there can be no doubt that psychiatrists sometimes identify with the parents' values and are too prone to label a rebellious child as a sick child. In such instances hospitalization may be unnecessary and potentially harmful to the child.

Two recent federal court decisions have attempted to deal with these problems by in effect providing children facing hospitalization with many of the same procedural rights as adults.[39] The constitutional arguments used to support these decisions are similar to those used in civil rights cases involving adult patients. The courts have noted a potential conflict of interest between the parents and the child, and have recommended that children facing hospitalization have such rights as a probable cause hearing, a full commitment hearing, a level of proof of clear and convincing evidence, and the right to counsel as well as mandatory use of counsel. In one federal case the state was ordered to proceed as expeditiously as possible to provide less restrictive or nonhospital facilities for the treatment of hospitalized children.[40] Both federal cases were appealed to the Supreme Court, which recently ruled that complex legal procedures for reviewing admission of children to hospitals are in most cases unnecessary. Review of the parents' request by a neutral physician, however, was felt to be constitutionally required.[41] This new ruling may lessen the problems of psychiatrists who treat hospitalized children, but it is still too early to predict its precise impact. The Court did not prohibit judicial review of children's hospitalization (it merely said it was unnecessary) and it did not deal with the issue of postadmission review procedures.

It is important to note that no U.S. court decisions have ruled that the involuntary hospitalization of children must be governed by procedures identical to those used with adults. Mental illness and need for treatment have consistently been viewed as sufficient criteria for hospitalization, and proof of dangerousness is not required. The reason for maintaining these relatively broad standards is recognition on the part of almost all interested parties that many children could not be expected to exercise sufficient judgment to enter the hospital voluntarily when they

---

[39]Parham v. J. L., 412 F. Supp. 112 (M.D. Ga.), *stay granted* 96 S. Ct. 1503 (1976), *probable jurisdiction noted,* 45 U.S.L.W. 3733 (May 31, 1979); and Bartley v. Kremens, 402 F. Supp. 1039 (E.D. Pa. 1975), *vacated and remanded,* 97 S. Ct. 1709, 45 U.S.L.W. 4451 (1977).

[40]Parham v. J. L., 412 F. Supp. 112 (M.D. Ga.), *stay granted* 96 S. Ct. 1503 (1976), *probable jurisdiction noted,* 45 U.S.L.W. 3733 (May 31, 1979).

[41]L. R. Roth, "Judicial Action Report," *Psychiatric News 14,* no. 17 (1979):

needed treatment. Since there would never be an opportunity for all admissions of children to be truly voluntary, the courts have not demanded that adult standards of involuntary commitment (dangerousness to self or others) be applied in situations where the child needs help but is unable to exercise the judgment to seek it willingly. Even with expanded due process a child can still be "voluntarily" hospitalized at the request of his parents if he is found to be mentally ill. All that is changed is that the child is given substantial procedural rights to protest this procedure.

What Are Some Problems Psychiatrists May Encounter in Dealing with Laws Which Expand Children's Rights to Resist Hospitalization?

For the most part our profession has recognized that abuses of children's rights can occur without court monitoring and has welcomed the expansion of procedural protections. Psychiatrists are concerned, however, as to whether the mandatory use of procedural safeguards is helpful to all children in all situations. One obvious concern is that judicial proceedings have different impacts on children of different ages. Judicial proceedings, for example, may not trouble an adolescent but may be quite harmful to a prepubertal child. Even though recent federal court rulings do provide that the competent child can waive a judicial hearing with the approval of his attorney, the prepubertal child may still be put under unusual stress and may have his chances of treatment compromised by consultation with an attorney who presents the child with an option of resisting the parents' wishes.[42]

Another obvious problem is that the new procedural rights are not based on an enlightened perspective of the differing problems of disturbed children. Children who are unruly and disobedient may or may not be mentally ill. They require protection of their civil rights. An adversarial proceeding may not be psychologically harmful to them and in some instances may help them. Children with psychoses and organic brain diseases, however, are unlikely to benefit from the process of legal definition of their illness status. They need a consistent, concerned, and compassionate adult world, and their encounter with an adversary process in which various adults publicly debate what is wrong with them can hardly be helpful.

A third major problem is that there is a great variation in the quality

[42]G. Planavsky, V. Ritchie, and Z. Silverstein, "Intensive Residential Treatment for Adolescents in North Carolina and the Present Legal System: A Review and Proposed Changes," *North Carolina Journal of Mental Health 8,* no. 9 (1978): 1–15.

of care provided by different treatment programs for children. Some are excellent and some are disgraceful. Elaborate procedural rights are absolutely necessary when the child faces confinement to an inadequate hospital setting. But these same processes may be harmful to the child and interfere with the kind of treatment that can be provided by an excellent program.

Since 1975 the state of North Carolina has by statute provided children most of the rights which have been sought in the federal courts.[43] The law still allows parents or guardians to admit a minor "voluntarily" to the hospital. To support such an admission the district court judge must determine only that the child is mentally ill and in need of care at a treatment facility. There is no dangerousness criterion. The law provides for most of the procedural rights available to adults including notice, counsel, and a postadmission hearing. The child must be interviewed and represented by a special counsel who is appointed as his lawyer, although the child can waive the right to appear at his hearing. It is unclear whether the special counsel functions as the child's advocate or functions solely in the child's best interests. This is a critical question since, as has been noted previously, the adolescent child's demand for freedom from hospitalization may be totally inconsistent with his best interests. The law also provides for rehearing at periodic intervals.

Those involved in some of the better treatment programs in North Carolina have noted that the procedures involved in this law can seriously interfere with the treatment needs of the child. The adversarial tone engendered by the initial hearing often interferes with the child's developing the kind of alliance with the treatment team that is necessary. Some children feel sentenced to the institution. Others who may have felt that they were at the institution on a truly voluntary basis are troubled by the court's clear expression that such is not the case. (These children may have wanted to hold onto their illusion of voluntariness.) The adversarial process may at times also make it difficult to impose necessary controls on disturbed children. As the court gains power to control the child's behavior, the institution loses it. The child may gear his behavior to pleasing the legal authorities and finding ways of gaining quick release, rather than being influenced by the institution's efforts to have him work on his problems. It has also been noted that attorneys who represent the child are likely to take the child's expressed wishes at face value. The child may view the attorney as his ally and the therapist as his adversary. When the child's demands to leave the hospital are really manifestations of anxiety and a need for control, and when the lawyer is pitted against the therapist in supporting the child's distur-

---

[43] *Ibid.*

bance, it becomes quite difficult for the child to make therapeutic progress.

In programs which involve long-term treatment of many months or years, the procedural issues are even more deleterious to treatment. Often after several months of treatment the child is much better, but is doing well primarily because he is institutionalized and is relying on the external controls of the hospital. Such a child who appears in court does not look mentally ill and the court has seriously to stretch the definition of mental illness in order to justify continued hospitalization. Sometimes it simply releases a child who is in no position to function outside the institution just at a time when treatment is becoming effective. It has also been speculated that some children who are doing well but who sense that they might be released and who fear such an outcome may deliberately engage in antisocial behavior or may escalate other symptoms in order to convince the court that they are indeed mentally ill and need to remain in the hospital.

As is the case with adults, it is probable that the new legal changes which protect civil rights of children will be of considerable help to those facing hospitalization in institutions which provide inferior care but may be harmful to those who have the opportunity to receive good care. Currently, there are more bad programs than good ones and it is difficult to foresee any radical improvement in children's institutions in the near future. Federal court decisions similar to the right to treatment decisions are currently having some impact on improving the levels of care for children confined to institutions for the mentally retarded.[44] But overall there is little reason to anticipate significant improvement of hospital facilities for mentally disturbed children throughout the nation. All this means that the need for safeguarding the rights of children in the mental health system will not go away even following the Supreme Court's decision to relax judicial review of children's hospitalizations.

Until the issue involving the rights of mentally disturbed children are finally litigated, psychiatrists have some opportunity to seek legislation which will serve the best interests of the child. It would seem useful that such legislation incorporate the following principles:

1. Hospital units which treat mentally disturbed children should be evaluated in terms of their staffing patterns and treatment facilities. Conceivably, standards of due process could be relaxed when children are hospitalized in institutions which have excellent facilities. It is conceivable that after an initial hearing a judge

[44]N.Y. State Association for Retarded Citizens and Parisi v. Carey, No. 72-C-356/357 (E.D. N.Y., April 30, 1975), *approved* 393 F. Supp. 715 (E.D. N.Y., 1975); P. R. Friedman, *The Rights of Mentally Retarded Persons* (New York: Avon Books, 1976).

or an impartial review committee could review the child's progress in an excellent institution without demanding rehearings.

2. In the case of prepubertal children who are hospitalized for relatively brief periods of time the entire adversarial process seems unnecessary. In this situation, an impartial review commission composed of attorneys, other interested citizens, and psychiatrists might simply review the hospitalization and progress of treatment.

3. All possible efforts should be made to develop standards for the care of hospitalized and emotionally disturbed children, and psychiatrists should assist in legal efforts to ascertain that these standards are implemented on a nationwide basis.

How Is Research with Human Subjects Regulated in Psychiatry?

Psychiatric research, like other forms of medical research, is subjected to regulation designed to protect the rights of human subjects. Courts may on occasion enunciate decisions which prohibit certain types of research, but for the most part experimentation is regulated by federal agencies which control funding to hospitals. Experimentation is also regulated to a lesser extent by malpractice law. Some doctors argue that any medical treatment is in effect a form of experimentation since there is always uncertainty of outcome. As a general rule, however, treatment is not defined as experimental unless there is considerable uncertainty as to outcome. In the usual definition of experimentation two elements are required: first, that the intervention be a departure from standard treatment; and second, that at least one of the purposes of the intervention be that of obtaining new knowledge for testing hypotheses. In some situations experimental interventions are used in the belief that they are of direct benefit to the patient (such as when a new drug is used to try to alleviate a serious disorder). In other instances the experiment may have little relevance to the patient's disturbance, but is designed to gain information about a disease or ultimately to help other patients. (An example here might be the testing of various physiological responses of schizophrenics to certain drugs.) Obviously, the second type of experiment needs more careful surveillance.

Almost all hospitals in the United States rely to some extent on HEW funds. To obtain these funds they must follow certain guidelines with regard to research. All research projects must be reviewed by a committee which consists of doctors who have no personal interest in the outcome of the research, as well as other professionals and interested citizens. In deciding whether to approve a research project the committee must consider three major issues: first, is the research sound? Second, are the benefits of the research intervention likely to outweigh its risks? And third, is there a true informed consent on the part of the patient?

As noted in a previous section there are three major elements to the doctrine of consent: voluntariness, competency, and knowledge. The issues with regard to knowledge are more or less similar in psychiatry and other branches of medicine. The issues of voluntariness and competency are somewhat different. Many psychiatric patients are subject to involuntary restraint which puts them in a somewhat subservient position toward doctors. The courts have seriously questioned whether individuals who are involuntarily deprived of freedom, either in prison or in hospitals, are really capable of "volunteering" for an experimental procedure.[45] It is assumed that the desire to please authorities may override the issue of voluntariness.

An even greater problem in psychiatric research is determining the competency of the patient. Some of the most important research in medicine must be done with the sickest patients. The sickest psychiatric patients are likely to be incompetent. As has been noted previously, the issue of competency is difficult to define and is most logically considered only in terms of specific functions. Standards of competency to consent to a treatment which has little risk and considerable likelihood of being beneficial are usually quite low. The tendency of the regulatory agency would be to find a given patient's consent in this situation to be competent. On the other hand the competency of a patient who consents to risky procedures is likely to be vigorously scrutinized. At the same time the patient who rejects risky treatments will not usually be viewed as incompetent, but those who reject treatments that are not risky and seem to be very much in their best interests are more likely to be adjudicated incompetent and might even be subjected to an experimental procedure through the consent of their guardians.

Parents can consent to experimental procedures for younger children when treatment benefits are likely and risks are minimal. With older children in similar situations it is advisable that the child and parents both consent after receiving full knowledge of the risks and benefits of treatment. When an experimental procedure provides no immediate benefit to the child and is risky, it will usually be prohibited or will be allowed only with court approval in addition to parental consent.

[45]Kaimowitz v. Michigan Department of Mental Health, Civil Action 73-19434-AW (Wayne County, Mich., Cir. Ct. 1973).

What Are Some Possible Consequences of the Continuation of Legal Control or Psychiatric Treatment of Severely Disturbed Patients?

One of the least defensible aspects of current psychiatric practice is the tendency of our profession (as well as other mental health professions) to focus most of its resources and efforts on patients who have the least severe illnesses. In other branches of medicine, as the patient gets sicker, the intensity and usually the quality of care increases. In psychiatry the opposite is true. The most skillful clinicians spend the largest amount of time working with the least disturbed. The most severely disturbed, even when they can afford good treatment, have difficulty finding it.

One explanation of this deplorable situation is that the rewards available to a psychiatrist in the way of money, status, and power are greatest when working with the least disturbed. State hospital psychiatrists who are likely to work with the most disturbed patients receive the least remuneration and have the least status and power within psychiatric organizations. In addition, work with severely disturbed patients is psychologically stressful, at times physically dangerous, and too often does not provide the physician with the reward of seeing the patient get well. Recruiting competent physicians to work in state hospital settings is an unremitting and practically unsolvable problem even under ordinary circumstances. The new legal control of psychiatry, however, will increase the difficulty of recruiting and keeping competent psychiatrists to treat severely disturbed patients.

The physician who elects to work in a state mental hospital these days must devote a considerable amount of time to legal issues. He is susceptible to lawsuits (on the basis of federal civil rights statutes) which are not covered by malpractice insurance. He must deal with the constant frustration of having the court terminate treatment of people who are obviously treatable. As a rule only the physician who has the least marketable skills will take such a job. The better doctors tend to get out at the first opportunity.

In effect, patients sent to mental hospitals these days are less likely to be treated by competent physicians than they were in past decades. Even if they are fortunate enough to find a competent physician, that doctor is likely to have less time to spend with them. They are also likely to encounter a doctor plagued with defensive attitudes and poor morale. The impact of the new legalism on psychiatric personnel then becomes translated into a deteriorated level of patient care.

The new laws have also created a large population of untreated mentally ill people who wander the streets of our cities. These individuals (whom Professor Slovenko describes as having been "railroaded" out of the hospital) suffer greatly, and they also impose a considerable burden on the community.[46] They are easily exploited by criminal elements within the society. They are usually incapable of making economic or social contributions to the community. Some commit minor crimes and end up in the criminal justice system. Here they are usually found incompetent to stand trial and are sent to hospitals for the criminally insane. (There tends to be some increase in commitments for incompetency to stand trial whenever the criteria for civil commitment become more stringent.)

We can expect the deterioration of health care for indigent severely disturbed patients to continue. As the public becomes hardened to the suffering of the mentally ill, they will view their presence in "mental illness ghettoes" as acceptable. City dwellers are becoming inured to a relatively noncompassionate lifestyle, and there seems to be little surge of public opinion demanding that the mentally ill within the community receive better care.

Another future scenario which is most depressing is the possibility that the right to refuse treatment will be sustained. We may then find our hospitals filled with people who are unlikely to get better. Some of these people will be violent toward other patients and personnel. Hospital units may once again become the "snake pits" they were before the availability of neuroleptic medication. One possible way in which hospitals might respond to such a situation would be to create separate wards for committed and voluntary patients. Separating committed (and perhaps "dangerous") patients who refuse treatment from voluntary and cooperative patients would at least provide a certain degree of protection to the latter group.

The most hopeful note in this whole area is that there has recently been an increased questioning of the usefulness of the standard of dangerousness in the civil commitment process. A federal court in 1978 ruled that the state of Illinois's present mental health code, which does not require an overt act of dangerousness to self or others for a person to be involuntarily civilly committed, is constitutional.[47] This was the first decision which seemed to go against the trend to require an increasing adherence to the protocols of the criminal law in the civil commitment process. Other states are now considering legislation which provides for broad enough definitions of dangerousness to allow for commitments of

[46]R. Slovenko and E. Luby, "From Moral Treatment to Railroading out of the Mental Hospital," *Bulletin of the American Academy of Psychiatry and the Law* 2, no. 4 (1977): 233–34.

[47]"U.S. Court upholds Danger Exam Standard," *Psychiatric News* 13, no. 13 (1978).

larger numbers of disabled persons. While modifications of the danger-ousness standard are not solutions to the problem of treating the se-verely disturbed, they provide some reason to hope that there is a new appreciation that the unreflective use of criminal justice procedures to resolve mental health problems is ultimately destructive.

9

Confidentiality in Psychiatric Practice

Effective diagnosis and treatment in psychiatry depend on the doctor's ability to collect information about the patient. This information is sometimes received directly from the patient, sometimes from medical records, and sometimes from the patient's friends or loved ones. Some of the information the doctor accumulates could be embarrassing and damaging to the patient if communicated to a third party. At the same time there are many instances in which sharing of information about the patient with others can be extremely beneficial to the patient. It is, therefore, critical that the psychiatric physician have guidelines to help him judge when he can pass on information about the patient to others. These guidelines should cover the regulation of information that is in the doctor's own head as well as in his medical records.

As previously noted, psychiatrists tend to be scrupulously concerned with harm that can result to the patient as a result of a betrayal of confidence. This concern is engrained in the consciousness of the psychiatrist from the first day of training. Much of the regulation of the flow of information in psychiatry is, therefore, self-regulation. Either the individual practitioner develops a system of internal guidelines or he relies on those of professional organizations. Much of the legal or external regulation of psychiatric information is controlled by tort law. The conditions under which a doctor can be sued for breach of confidentiality, defamation, and invasion of privacy have been discussed in Part I. In this chapter the emphasis will be on the manner in which the flow of information about the patient is influenced by federal regulatory agencies, by statutory law, and by ethical considerations.

Information about the patient can be requested by the patient, by the patient's relatives, by the courts, by public welfare agencies, by employers and licensing agencies, by insurance companies, and by a variety of private and public agencies which reimburse the physician or the hospital for treatment of the patient. Each of these individuals or agencies may request information for the purpose of helping the patient or for purposes which help someone other than the patient. In the latter instance, sharing of information may harm rather than benefit the patient. Occasionally individuals seeking information about the patient may intend to use that information to hurt the patient.

What Problems Can Arise in Releasing Information about a Psychiatric Patient to Other Persons Involved in the Patient's Treatment?

In the hospital setting all people involved in the patient's treatment should receive as much information about the patient as they need to carry out their treatment task. There is usually no problem when the psychiatrist shares information with nurses, social workers, or recreational and occupational therapists. If the psychiatrist calls in consultants, of course, there must be free exchange of information between the referring doctor and the consultant. There are probably a few situations in which communication with colleagues and the treatment team might be limited. The prudent psychiatrist will exercise some restraint in determining whether information that is not relevant to the patient's treatment and which may be embarrassing to the patient should be put in medical records or communicated to colleagues and other helping professionals. Certain kinds of material involving atypical sexual behavior, for example, may be highly embarrassing to the patient, and if such information is not relevant to the treatment process it is probably best that it not be recorded or shared with others.

When the patient is referred to another doctor and the patient has signed a release or waiver from which acknowledges the patient's wish to have the new doctor receive past records, it is customary for the psychiatrist to release as much information as is requested to the new doctor. There is usually no problem involved when the new doctor is simply involved in continuing the process of treatment. Often, however, such requests are made by doctors who are employed by agencies. Information here may be used to make decisions as to whether to employ an individual, insure him, or grant him some privilege such as entry into a university. The doctor requesting information may be more concerned with the needs of his organization than with the needs of the patient.[1] Releasing information in this situation is similar to releasing information directly to an agency. Even though it is a colleague who is requesting information, the psychiatrist should try to ascertain that the patient has signed a competent and informed waiver before the requested material is released.

Telephone calls from other doctors requesting information should be handled with special caution. Unless the psychiatrist knows the calling person, he has no reassurance that the caller is really who he says he is. Even when the psychiatrist has good reason to believe that the caller actually is a physician, he should still be wary of releasing information without the patient's authorization. Unfortunately, there are some doctors who have a responsibility to an agency who will call the treating psychiatrist (or will appear in his office) and "as one doctor to another" will request information about the patient without the benefit of the patient's knowledge or consent. A university hospital psychiatrist, for example, will not infrequently receive requests for information about patients from other doctors responsible for the health of hospital employees or university students. Although the psychiatrist may not enhance his professional image by refusing to divulge information to other doctors, he should be steadfast in refusing to release information to an agency-employed colleague without the patient's written consent.

Requests of other physicians for information which the patient has not authorized to be released may have a special urgency in situations where the patient has some responsible job (for example, as a police officer or commercial pilot) which may involve public safety. Here the psychiatrist is usually wise to urge the patient to authorize release of information when the agency doctor requests it. In most instances the patient's possible threat to the safety of others will not be nearly as grave as the agency fears and communication of factual material might put everyone at ease. If the patient does have a problem which represents a serious threat to public safety (for example, a commercial airline pilot who is abusing alcohol), the doctor has an ethical obligation to do something about the situation. If the patient refuses to authorize release of information and the psychiatrist firmly believes that the patient is (like the airline pilot) in a position to hurt others, the psychiatrist should not balk at telling the agency-employed physician about the problem or should report the problem directly to the physician even before any request for information is made. Such violation of the patient's confiden-

---

[1] W. H. Van Hoose and J. A. Kottler, *Ethical and Legal Issues in Counseling and Psychotherapy,* (San Francisco: Jossey-Bass, 1977).

tiality may go against our training and inclinations, but our obligations to the welfare of others makes it morally and legally justifiable.

What Legal Issues Are Involved in Allowing Patients Access to Their Own Records?

The courts usually assume that the patient's outpatient or hospital records are the property of the physician, but that the information which they contain should be controlled by the patient.[2] The patient, however, even in nonpsychiatric medicine, usually has considerable difficulty in gaining access to his own records. There may be good reasons for the patient's wanting to examine his record. An informed patient who has no secrets kept from him can relate to the physician in a more egalitarian manner and is unlikely to feel patronized or infantilized by his doctor. The patient may want access to something in his record to clarify issues that would help him in a lawsuit or in efforts to obtain Workmen's Compensation or some form of government service. It is also possible in this day and age when so many agencies have access to the patient's record, and there is reason to worry about who is actually reading a record, that the patient might want to correct something in the chart that was inaccurate and that others might use to harm him.

There is certainly a good case for allowing nonpsychiatric patients the right of access to their records. It is likely that this right will be vigorously pursued by patients and their advocates, and the day is probably not too far away when all patients will have complete or considerable access to their own records. At the present time, however, the law in this area is very unclear and varies from state to state. In most states the patient can obtain access to his records only by consenting to have them released to another physician or to the patient's attorney. The new physician or the attorney may then be willing to share the contents of the record with the patient. In states where the law is more liberal some hospitals and doctors are allowing patients to examine their own records. Even psychiatric patients are granted this right in most circumstances.

Whatever the laws of a particular state might be, there are certain situations in which it might be nontherapeutic or harmful to the psychiatric patient to examine his own record. Reading about the severity of his illness and his actual behavior while sick might both frighten and humiliate the patient. If the patient is still emotionally disturbed, he can seriously misinterpret the contents of the record and become upset

---

[2]G. Annas, *The Rights of Hospital Patients* (New York: Avon Books, 1975), chap. 10.

and moved to take inappropriate actions. Sometimes misinterpretation of material in the chart may compromise the patient's motivation to continue in needed treatment. In most states the psychiatrist still holds the power to withhold records from patients whom he believes should not see them, and it is likely that even with changes in other specialties of medicine a limited degree of this power will probably be retained in psychiatry.

What Legal Issues Must the Psychiatrist Consider in Releasing Information to Relatives of the Patient?

There are few statutes or precedents in this area, and for the most part the psychiatrist's behavior will be guided by ethical considerations and concern over possible breaches of confidentiality that might result in malpractice suits. Relatives are likely to have entirely benevolent motivations in seeking information about their loved one, but this is not always the case. Spouses may want to use information about their husband's or wife's illness in a divorce suit or in a child custody case. Parents as well as spouses may use psychiatric information to control, belittle, or humiliate the patient. As has been noted in the section on malpractice, the psychiatrist must use considerable discretion in revealing information to relatives, and the patient's confidentiality should be honored to the fullest extent possible. The safest and most ethical practice is to reach an agreement with the patient as to what information he wishes to have shared with relatives. (For a more detailed discussion of this issue, the reader is referred to the section on breach of confidentiality in Part I.)

What Legal Issues Are Involved When the Courts Ask the Psychiatrist for Information about a Patient He Has Treated?

Certain communications between two parties, one of whom is in a professional relationship to the other, are judged to be privileged in the sense that the professional person cannot reveal these communications even in the courtroom. This is true of the priest–penitent relationship or the attorney–client relationship. In the above examples such privilege has long been available through the common law.[3] This testimonial privilege can be viewed as an exception to the usual obligation of any citizen to testify when called upon to do so by a court. The exception

[3]R. Slovenko, *Psychiatry and Law* (Boston: Little, Brown, 1973), chap. 4.

arises from the assumption that certain relationships depend on free communication and are so special and significant that the protection of that free communication is more important than the needs of government for truth and relevant fact.

Historically the testimonial privilege as a shield against access to facts that might be sought by the court has been granted only in limited situations involving lawyers and clients or clergymen and penitents. There is no privilege in the common law protecting the patient's communication to doctors. Privilege in the doctor–patient relationship did not develop in this country until this century and is almost wholly determined by statutory law. The first medical privilege statute in this country was enacted in New York in 1928, and its purpose was to help in the control of communicable diseases.[4] It was assumed that the possibility of embarrassment or disgrace that might result from eventual court disclosure of the fact of having such illnesses might deter some individuals from seeking and obtaining needed medical treatment. Many states have since followed the lead of New York and have enacted similar privilege statutes for physicians. Communications to psychiatrists, as physicians, are, therefore, deemed to be privileged in most jurisdictions. Recently a number of states have extended this privilege to relationships between nonphysician psychotherapists and patients.[5]

Testimonial privilege is never absolute. There are statutory limits on privilege and sometimes the court's or society's overriding "need to know" which exists independent of statutory law is regarded as more important than the maintenance of the patient's confidentiality. Any citizen, for example, regardless of his relationship with a patient or client, has a duty to communicate to law enforcement officials the knowledge of the imminent commission of a serious crime. There are still other limitations on statutory privilege which are extensive enough so that some have argued that they make the concept of privilege almost nonfunctional.[6] Privilege is usually forfeited when a patient injects his condition into litigation, arguing that the condition is an element which should support his claim or should help him in his defense. If the patient introduces his mental condition in his claim and his psychiatrist has knowledge of that condition, the psychiatrist may be asked to testify. Communications to the physician also lose privileged status in proceedings involving involuntary hospitalization. Here it is assumed that the interests of both the patient and society require a waiver of confidential-

---

[4] *Ibid.*

[5] C. Kennedy, "The Psychotherapists' Privilege," *Washburn Law Journal 12,* no. 3 (1973): 297–316.

[6] "Therapeutic Confidentiality," *Mental Disability Law Reporter 2,* no. 2–3 (1977): 339.

ity. Another important area in which privilege may be waived involves child custody hearings where society's regard for the "best interests of the child" leads the courts to demand full disclosure.

It is important to note that the privilege belongs to the patient and not to the doctor. It is the patient who waives his privilege by injecting his mental condition into the litigation as a claim or defense. The doctor is then in a passive position where he may be required to testify. Some psychiatrists have a great deal of difficulty in accepting this concept. They feel that the patient may be psychologically damaged by having details of his case revealed in court. They reason that just because the patient has made a bad judgment by injecting his mental condition into the litigation, the psychiatrist should not cooperate in what can be seen as a breach of confidentiality that may ultimately damage the patient. In two California cases in which patients injected their mental condition as a factor in tort cases their psychiatrists challenged the waiver of privilege provision of the California statutes by refusing to comply with the court's request to testify. Both went to jail briefly for contempt of court. In the ultimate resolution of the first case, the California court held that while a psychiatrist had no independent claim to the privilege and that it belonged to the patient, the psychiatrist's records and reports would be carefully screened by the court to determine what contents were or were not relevant to the case at hand and that only relevant material would be admitted into evidence.[7] To some psychiatrists this seemed to be a fair ruling, but it did not assuage the concerns of a second psychiatrist who was not convinced that his information could be screened by the courts in a manner that fully protected his patient. This doctor argued that an independent examination of the patient by impartial psychiatrists would provide the information required by the courts. His proposal, however, was not accepted and he was found in contempt.[8] In a more recent case a psychiatrist was asked by the court to reveal information about a woman in treatment who was involved in a child custody case. The patient in this case refused to grant permission for her records to be disclosed, but did agree to be examined by a court-selected psychiatrist. The psychiatrist refused to testify, was held in contempt of court, and then challenged the court's ruling. He was vindicated by the Pennsylvania Supreme Court in a closely divided ruling.[9] The court in this case based its decision on a constitutional right to privacy and gave the decision a breadth which one authority hopes will provide a degree of

[7]A. H. Bernstein, "Protecting Psychiatric Records," *Hospitals* 47 (1973): 100–103.
[8]"Psychiatrist Jailed in Privilege Challenge," *Psychiatric News* 12, no. 16 (1977): 1.
[9]R. Sadoff, "Pennsylvania Psychiatrist Vindicated in Refusing Judge's Request for Records," *Legal Aspects of Medical Practice* 7, no. 2 (1979): 38–39.

privilege to doctors and patients similar to that granted in lawyer–client relationships.[10] It is likely that if the Pennsylvania Supreme Court's example is followed by other jurisdictions, the doctor–patient privilege will be less governed by statute than by constitutional law and will have fewer restrictions. Most psychiatrists would probably like to see some of the exceptions to testimonial privilege removed, especially in situations like that in the Pennsylvania case where the patient was still in therapy and was strongly opposed to revealing therapy-generated information about herself in court. This is one legal area in which the psychiatrist has the opportunity to make personal sacrifices to bring about social change. The amount of risk a psychiatrist will want to take in defying a court order and risking a contempt citation, however, will depend on the details of a given case and the psychiatrist's own commitment to the concept of privilege.

Under What Circumstances Is the Psychiatrist Expected to Make Unauthorized Disclosures about the Patient to Regulatory Agencies?

In most states there are statutes which require the psychiatrist to report child abuse. The patient has no privilege when information regarding abuse or neglect of children is revealed. Doctors in many states may be required to report gunshot wounds, acute poisoning, motor vehicle accidents, or venereal diseases. When the doctor learns that a crime is to be committed, and particularly when the therapist firmly believes there is an imminent, clear, and substantial risk of the patient's hurting someone, the psychiatrist has at least an ethical obligation to break confidentiality either by initiating commitment, by warning police officers, or by warning the third party. In California under the special conditions described previously under *Tarasoff*, the psychiatrist may have a legal duty to warn third parties in danger.

What Legal and Ethical Issues Are Involved When the Psychiatrist Deals with Requests for Information about a Patient from Employers, Life Insurance Companies, or Licensing Boards?

Until quite recently, applicants for federal jobs were required to state whether they had received previous psychiatric treatment. Such information is still requested by many employers. It is routinely requested by insurance companies which insure for health, death benefits, or income protection. Licensing boards, whether regulating licenses to

[10]"State Court Upholds Records' Privilege," *Psychiatric News 13*, no. 12 (1978): 1.

drive an automobile or to practice professions such as law and medicine, may also ask the applicant if he has ever received psychiatric treatment. As a rule, if the job seeker or the insurance or licensing applicant reveals that he has received treatment, he is asked to sign a consent form which allows the company or agency to request information from the doctor who has treated the patient. If the patient does not authorize such release of information he is unlikely to receive the job, the policy, or the license.

The psychiatrist who must respond to these requests for information is in a difficult ethical situation. He is at no legal risk in releasing information as long as the patient has signed a proper authorization form. But the things he may have to say about the patient could end up hurting the patient. Even though the patient's psychiatric difficulties may have no relevance to the question of employability, insurability, or licensing, they may be used as grounds for denying the patient's requests. Psychiatrists have taken a variety of different ethical positions on this issue. Some refuse to send any information at all, although there is always a risk that this will hurt the patient. Most will refuse to release all their records, but will generally send a letter which answers the specific questions asked about the patient. It is probable that many psychiatrists will "fudge" in this situation and only reveal "good" things about the patient. Of course, a psychiatrist who did this consistently would soon lose all credibility with the information-requesting agencies. Other psychiatrists simply respond to the request as honestly as possible and never know which patients are hurt in the process. There is really no satisfactory way of dealing with this problem.

There is a major clinical issue here which may one day have legal implications. When the patient comes for therapy he usually expects full confidentiality and does not anticipate that someday he may be in a position where in order to get a job, a policy, or a license he must reveal the fact of his having been in therapy and thereby sacrifice confidentiality. The patient, in effect, is unlikely to know about one of the risks of treatment, namely, that his confidentiality can be violated with resulting embarrassment and loss of opportunity. This risk is relevant to the doctrine of informed consent. It would make sense for all psychotherapists to inform patients before therapy begins that third parties might someday wish to know facts as to the patient's disorder and treatment, that the patient may not be in a position to control release of this information, and that there is a certain risk that the psychiatrist's response may end up depriving the patient of something he wants.[11]

In the fifteen years in which I directed a student health psychiatry

[11]R. Sadoff, "Informed Consent, Confidentiality and Privilege in Psychiatry: Practical Applications," *Bulletin of the American Academy of Psychiatry and the Law* 2, no. 2 (1974): 1.

service I dealt with many requests for information from third parties. In the great majority of instances the kind of material available in the student's records had no relevance whatsoever to the purposes for which it was being requested. Often many years had elapsed since the patient had been treated and there was no way of knowing anything at all about the patient's mental status at the time information was requested. It always seemed most reasonable to me that if an employer wanted to know if an applicant was too impaired to do a certain type of work that the employer could hire his own psychiatrist who would know something about the kind of job for which the patient was being considered and who could interview the applicant and make a rational and timely assessment of his capacity to handle the job. Similar considerations would apply to insurance policies and licenses. The agency-employed psychiatrist would be identified clearly as being in a role that required dual allegiances. He might want to help the patient, but his primary obligation would be to his employer. He would have no illusions as to his double-agent role, and would, in fairness, warn the patient of the possible adverse recommendations which might arise from the examination. Under such a system the patient would have no sense of being vulnerable because of past therapy, no sense of being spied on, and no fear of "betrayal" by his therapist. The above system of evaluation would be fair to all parties, but its relative expense has probably curtailed its usage. Most agencies continue to seek the questionably useful, but certainly less expensive, means of getting information by contacting the patient's previous doctor.

What Are Some of the Legal and Ethical Issues Involved in Divulging Information to Insurance Companies and Federal Agencies Which Pay for Health Care?

As third-party payment through private insurance companies or government agencies has become common in medical practice, it has also created a serious problem with regard to the issue of confidentiality. Private insurers as well as the public are extremely cost conscious. As the cost of health care rises there is a great demand for accountability and claims for hospital and doctors' bills must be justified. As noted in the section on malpractice, fraud on the part of the doctor is possible in dealing with third-party payers, and one way of controlling fraud is by careful surveillance of the process of diagnosis and treatment. Obviously, private insurance companies and federal agencies have powerful motivations for seeking information regarding patient care, and the growth of the third-party payment has inevitably led to a certain erosion of confidentiality.[12]

The need for third-party payers as well as other groups involved in the health care process to have access to information about patients has also led to the development of centralized computer banks where a great deal of medical and psychiatric information about an individual can be stored. Centralized computers offer some advantages to the patient. They make quickly retrievable and legible information available in whatever part of the country the patient is being treated. They also facilitate the gathering of medical statistics and epidemiological studies. The problem with centralized computerization of medical information, however, is that it increases the risk that unauthorized persons may gain access to patient information. This can happen through theft or through careless handling of files.

Psychiatrists are deeply concerned with threats of confidentiality related to third-party payments and computerization of records. Currently there are several national commissions trying to work out guidelines to provide maximum protection to patients within a system which requires so much monitoring of information.[13] Some of the urgency in this area is fueled by periodic reports of gross misuse of data about psychiatric patients. In various instances, unauthorized information has ended up in the hands of employers, educational institutes, police, credit bureaus, and government licensing agencies. Our urgency is also related to the realization that problems of maintaining confidentiality will increase massively if and when national health insurance becomes a reality.

At this point we are far from clear as to how we can meet social needs for accountability while still preserving the rights of patients. Two relatively minor innovations have been suggested, however, which should not interfere too much with agency needs, but which should help patients. One is that consent forms which patients sign and which allow for release of information to third parties should state with some precision exactly what information can be released and what cannot. Currently many of the forms allow for release of all available information, much of which is not relevant to the question of reimbursement. The so-called blanket consent form is a threat to the patient's privacy which can be substantially reduced. A second recommendation is that

[12]P. Chodoff, "Psychiatry and the Fiscal Third Party," *American Journal of Psychiatry 135*, no. 10 (1978): 1141–47; American Psychiatric Association, "Confidentiality and Third Parties: A Report of the APA Task Force on Confidentiality as It Relates to Third Parties" (Washington, D.C.: APA, 1975).

[13]See "Health Records and Confidentiality, An Annotated Bibliography with Abstracts" (Washington, D.C.: National Commission on Confidentiality of Health Records, 1977).

patients have unrestricted access to computerized health information so that they are in a position to correct errors.[14]

Are There Special Legal Problems Involving Confidentiality in Group and Family Therapy?

There are no legal precedents regarding control of information in group therapy. This does not mean that psychiatrists have been unaware of serious ethical questions regarding confidentiality in groups and do not fear future litigation. Many group therapists feel that they are sitting on a legal and ethical volcano.[15] Obviously patients in group therapy might gossip about each other and there is little that can be done to control this. Conceivably the patient could be damaged by this breach of confidentiality and might have a cause of action against other group members or the therapist. Thus far, however, there has been no litigation involving breach of confidentiality in groups. Nor is there any litigation which raises the question of whether information generated in the group is privileged. One legal scholar has questioned whether privilege would disappear if a member of the group sued another or if a group member involved in some process of litigation raised his mental health as a claim or defense in the judicial process.[16] Other kinds of speculation regarding disclosure of information in group therapy can be made such as whether or not group members in the state of California might, under *Tarasoff*, have some obligation to warn third parties of threats of violence made in the course of therapy.

There has been a small amount of litigation as to whether information generated in family therapy is privileged. Problems can arise when spouses receive conjoint treatment and are subsequently involved in divorce or child custody proceedings. Family members who are parties to litigation involving one another are, of course, free to use information they recall hearing in the course of conjoint psychotherapy. But thus far the courts have ruled that any records which may have been kept, as well as any testimony based on the psychiatrist's recollection of what was revealed in the course of therapy, are privileged.[17] The granting of

[14]G. J. Annas, *The Rights of Mental Patients* (New York: Avon Books 1975), chap. 10.

[15]L. Foster, "Group Psychotherapy: A Pool of Legal Witnesses," *International Journal of Group Psychotherapy* 25 (1975): 50.

[16]R. Slovenko, "Group Psychotherapy: Privileged Communication and Confidentiality," *Journal of Psychiatry and Law,* fall, 1977, pp. 405–67.

[17]Ellis v. Ellis, 472 S.W.2d 741 (Tenn. Aff. 1971); but a more recent case suggests that this issue is far from settled: see "Privilege Denied in Joint Therapy," *Psychiatric News 14,* no. 9 (1979): 1.

complete privilege in family therapy, particularly couple therapy, makes sense since people who enter such treatment are usually having difficulties with one another and the risk of their becoming involved in divorce or child custody litigation is far greater than average. Fewer of these people would be willing to seek the benefits of therapy if they feared that subsequent disclosure of what was revealed would embarrass them or compromise the strength of their case in subsequent litigation.

PART III
EXPERT WITNESS ROLES

10

General Issues Regarding Psychiatric Testimony

In resolving some types of legal conflicts the court may seek information as to the mental status of one or more of the litigants. Often this information will have a critical influence on the court's decision. The legal system uses the testimony and observations of ordinary persons in determining certain aspects of a litigant's mental status such as his motivation. However, the presence of most forms of mental impairment is usually determined with the assistance of experts. The psychiatrist is commonly asked to evaluate litigants and testify as to their mental status. He can provide facts (such as the existence of abnormal laboratory tests) that would not otherwise be available to the court. He can also provide professional opinions as to the litigant's emotional status. These will be respected by the court and will be given more weight than the testimony of ordinary persons.

The psychiatrist who involves himself in expert witness roles comes to court voluntarily. He knows (or should know) that there are some minor risks involved in his participation. He also knows that the benefits of the expert role can be substantial. The expert witness is usually paid for his participation (these days, sometimes quite handsomely), receives considerable emotional support and praise from at least one of the parties in the adversary process, and may also be pleasantly distracted from the tedium of everyday practice. Sometimes the psychiatrist as an expert witness may feel that his testimony helps to support a social position which he firmly advocates. Here the expert witness is in the happy position of being able to make money and further his moral and political beliefs at the same time. As an expert witness, the psychiatrist clearly receives more gratification in his encounters with the courts than when he is a defendant in a malpractice case or when he must go to court to find a legally acceptable way to treat a disturbed patient. There are now several hundred psychiatrists who devote much of their professional practice to testifying as experts. This field has grown so rapidly that a new accrediting board in legal psychiatry has recently been created.

Some psychiatrists become involved in the role of expert witness as a part of their job in state mental health or criminal justice facilities. A doctor who works for a mental hospital, a community clinic, a court clinic, or a hospital for the criminally insane may be required to testify in court as to whether a given patient was insane at the time he was alleged to have committed a crime, is currently incompetent to stand trial, or currently meets the requirements for civil commitment. (The role of the court-appointed and state-employed examiner in the civil commitment process is most appropriately viewed as that of an expert witness. Of course, the examining psychiatrist who recommends civil commitment can later turn out to be the person who is responsible for the committed patient's treatment.) Psychiatrists in private practice become involved as experts when they respond to requests for their services by the state or the defendant in criminal cases or by the plaintiff or defendant in civil cases. The psychiatrist who works in a community where there are many practitioners can usually avoid expert witness roles and leave them to colleagues with greater forensic interests. Psychiatrists who live in communities which do not have a high concentration of colleagues, however, may be the only experts available and should be prepared to participate in a large variety of cases. A psychiatrist can also find himself in an expert role through unanticipated circumstances. Sometimes a patient already in treatment may ask the psychiatrist to help him with a legal problem by testifying as to his mental status. The problem may have little to do with the patient's treatment needs and in some instances the patient may be helped by honoring his request.

The major areas in which psychiatrists are asked to perform as expert witnesses in the criminal courts involve the determination of an offender's possible lack of guilt by reason of insanity and an offender's competency or incompetency to stand trial. More recently, psychiatrists have been asked to provide expert testimony which is directed toward clarifying mitigating or aggravating circumstances in cases where the death penalty might be invoked. Psychiatrists, of course, are also involved in the legal process as educators, as therapists of offenders, and as consultants who assist in the disposition of offenders through various stages of the criminal justice process. These latter roles, although extremely important, are rarely assumed by the ordinary practitioner, however, and do not require courtroom testimony; thus, they will not be discussed here. In civil courts the psychiatrist may assume an expert witness role in determining an individual's need for civil commitment (already discussed), in making recommendations regarding child custody, in assessing psychic injury, in determining an individual's competency to participate in a variety of social functions, in malpractice cases, and in litigation influencing the civil rights of various classes of people.

As a general rule, the psychiatrist testifies as a partisan witness who is employed by one side or another in the adversary system. Sometimes, however, the state-employed psychiatrist is the only expert witness available. This is often the case in civil commitment and criminal justice proceedings. In these situations the psychiatrist is presumed to be an impartial witness whose main purpose is to serve the court and whose reports and conclusions are available to both the prosecution and the defense.

The psychiatrist can also become involved in the litigation process in the role of *amicus curiae*, or friend of the court. As a rule, the court will allow individuals or organizations to introduce arguments or evidence in suits to which they are not a party, but the outcome of which is likely to affect them. In addition to protecting his own interest, the *amicus curiae* may call the attention of the court to relevant legal issues it is in danger of disregarding. While the *amicus curiae* brief is usually presented by an attorney, the psychiatrist can provide considerable input into the content of the brief and in effect introduce his views to the court. Increasingly, interested parties have volunteered to be friends of the court and lobby for their position in major cases involving broad social issues. Suits involving the rights of patients have elicited considerable attention from professional mental health organizations. The American Orthopsychiatric Association has been especially active in taking positions in cases involving civil commitment and competency to stand trial. The American Psychiatric Association has been somewhat reluctant to get into the *amicus curiae* role, but it now has a commission on judicial action which provides expert briefs in cases which may have general impact on the practice of psychiatry whether these cases involve civil rights or malpractice actions.

Although the field of forensic psychiatry is expanding and although more and more psychiatrists are willing to serve as expert witnesses, it must be noted that a large number of psychiatrists avoid courtroom involvement like the plague. There are multiple reasons for this. Some psychiatrists are uncomfortable with or intolerant of the adversarial approach to truth finding. They distrust attorneys and want to have as little to do with them as possible. Other psychiatrists fear the anxiety and feelings of powerlessness which are inherent risks of exposure to cross-examination. Moral or ideological committments may also keep psychiatrists out of the courtroom.[1] Many psychiatrists, perhaps even

---

[1]J. Robitscher and R. Williams, "Should Psychiatrists Get Out of the Courtroom?" *Psychology Today*, December 1977. R. Leifer, *In the Name of Mental Health* (New York: Science House, 1966).

the majority, feel that they have nothing to contribute to determining a person's guilt by reason of insanity or a person's competency to stand trial. Nor are they convinced that their participation as experts in civil matters is either necessary or useful. They see little reason to anticipate that the testimony provided by the psychiatrist will ultimately contribute to the improvement of society, and in some instances fear that psychiatric testimony can help perpetuate an oppressive status quo. Other psychiatrists believe that the standards by which they are required to testify, such as the standard of dangerousness, require responses beyond their expertise and that they cannot answer the questions which the court asks without perjuring themselves. Still others refuse to become involved in malpractice cases because they do not wish to speak poorly of colleagues or harm them. Finally, many psychiatrists (and certainly many jurists) are troubled by the manner in which expert psychiatric testimony tends to be primarily available to the affluent.[2] The indigent litigant must either rely on an impartial expert (usually a state-employed psychiatrist whose impartiality may be compromised by allegiances to the community which employs him) or none at all. The affluent litigant can afford to search for and hire a psychiatrist who is sympathetic to his position. Psychiatrists may decide to refuse to perpetuate these inequities by refusing to become involved as hired witnesses.

To What Extent Is the Psychiatrist Truly an Adversary When He Is Hired by One Side or Another in a Judicial Dispute?

There is considerable agreement among psychiatrists who do a lot of courtroom work that a psychiatrist can comfortably sustain a truly adversarial role only until he is actually sworn as a witness. In preparing his report, in reviewing the attorney's case, in anticipating cross-examination, and in anticipating and contradicting testimony of other expert witnesses, the psychiatrist can fully commit himself to the cause of his employer. If the psychiatrist enjoys competition, he can exercise all his skills and talents in helping the attorney present the strongest possible case and making the strongest possible use of the psychiatrist's own testimony. The psychiatrist who is committed to using the expert witness role to help initiate social change may up to this point allow himself similar indulgence. Once the psychiatrist is sworn in, however, and takes the witness stand, he should cease to view himself as an adversary. At this point he becomes a servant of the court. This point cannot be overstressed. The psychiatrist when testifying must have the

[2]S. L. Halleck, *The Politics of Therapy* (New York: Science House, 1971).

psychological flexibility to initiate a modest change in his identity. (The mental mechanism involved here is dissociation. In this instance the defense is used solely in the service of the ego.) When he takes the witness stand the psychiatrist becomes a person committed to the process of truth seeking no matter how the truth may conflict with his own ideologies. At this point the psychiatrist should not be reluctant to reveal information that may be adverse to his client's interest. He should never make any effort to embellish his testimony in a manner which leads to even minor distortions of information.

The psychiatrist's abandonment of the adversarial role when taking the witness stand should put him in a very comfortable position. Once the thought of "winning the case" is temporarily dissociated from his consciousness, the psychiatrist has no duty other than that of telling what he knows as clearly as possible. He emerges as a sincere and honorable witness. He is not likely to be riled by vigorous cross-examination, but rather can view such interrogation as a welcome technique for bringing out the strengths and shortcomings of his testimony. The psychiatrist who forgets he is no longer an adversary when he takes the witness stand risks becoming an inferior witness who can easily be embarrassed or humiliated in the course of testimony.

How Does the Psychiatrist Prepare to Testify as an Expert Witness?

The state-employed psychiatrist who is asked to serve as an expert by the court is usually quite familiar with the particular role he is asked to fill. It is unlikely that he will be asked to appear in more than one or two roles and he quickly learns to deal with the demands they make on him. The situation is different for the private practitioner who may be asked to respond to a variety of issues, and he may have little familiarity with any of them. The following advice is directed toward the private practitioner. The first thing to do is to clarify the issue about which testimony is being requested. The psychiatrist needs to know the precise nature of the conflict being adjudicated, the facts of the case, and the standards to which he will be asked to direct his testimony. It is important at this point also to establish ground rules. The psychiatrist's fee should be negotiated in as businesslike a manner as possible.

Here it is important to note that the psychiatrist is paid for his time. Courtroom testimony may make unusual demands on the doctor's time. The psychiatrist must be prepared to charge not only for the time he spends examining the patient but should also charge for time spent discussing the case with attorneys, for preparing reports, for being in court, and for testifying on the witness stand. Charging a flat fee is usually unwise since the amount of time likely to be spent on a given case is unpredictable. In criminal cases where the defendant may be convicted and sent to prison, the psychiatrist may wish to protect his financial interests by collecting a retainer in advance.

The conditions under which the patient will be examined must be clarified. It is essential that the psychiatrist ascertain that the patient will be available at certain times and in appropriate settings where competent interviewing is possible. He should also ascertain that all medical and legal records will be available, that access to other witnesses can be available on request, and that consultation with other nonpsychiatric physicians and the opportunity to do psychological and other testing are also available.

The qualifications of the psychiatric witness establishes expertise. These will usually be introduced in court and it is best that the attorney elicit these qualifications question by question. If the psychiatrist is simply asked to list his own qualifications, he may appear pompous. It is important that the attorney be provided with a copy of the psychiatrist's curriculum vitae so that he knows the expert's qualifications and can methodically introduce them to the court at the time of trial.

It is essential that the psychiatrist have a pretrial conference with the attorney or attorneys. The court-appointed psychiatrist may consult with both the defense attorney and district attorney. The partisan witness, however, will usually be asked to review his testimony only with the attorney who has hired him. It is important that he point out its strengths and weaknesses. He should, where possible, advise the attorney as to instances in which he believes the testimony is vulnerable to cross-examination. The psychiatrist can also use the pretrial conference to review the legal issues in controversy and check again to see that his planned testimony will be relevant to the case.

What Steps Should the Psychiatrist Take in Examining the Patient and Preparing a Report for the Court?

It is wise to begin by reviewing all the available medical and legal records. In instances involving criminal conduct, it is also useful to review police reports. At the time of the first interview, the patient should receive an explicit statement as to the psychiatrist's role in the examination and subsequent legal proceedings. This explanation should be sufficiently detailed so that the patient has a clear idea of the various ways in which the psychiatrist's report can either be consistent with or antagonistic to the patient's interest. The amount of time spent examining the patient will depend on the type of issue being considered, logistical issues such as the patient's and the doctor's availability, and the clinical style of the psychiatrist. Some psychiatrists believe they can do a relatively thorough evaluation in one or two hours. Most require much more time. It should be obvious that the more time the psychiatrist spends in examining the patient, the more likely he is to obtain accurate and comprehensive information and the more likely is he to impress the court with his testimony. There are, of course, patients who are relatively noncommunicative and for whom extended evaluation will not expand the available data base significantly. Most patients, however, should be interviewed for several hours. The psychiatrist should also feel free to utilize whatever tests may be helpful in evaluating the patient and in answering the legal questions involved in the case.

The psychiatrist will want to keep notes during the course of the examination which will assist him in organizing his eventual testimony. In some instances, particularly when the psychiatrist is an impartial expert, he may be asked to submit a report which may be examined by both the prosecuting and defense attorneys. These reports should be as thorough and jargon free as possible. Like the psychiatrist's actual testimony in court, they should focus on the data from which the psychiatrist derived his opinion. (For legal procedural reasons, the psychiatrist who prepares a report may not be able to read it on the stand. He may, however, refer to it or any other notes or records when presenting testimony.)

Finally, the psychiatrist should remind himself repeatedly that it is always the court which must make decisions as to the legal issue in controversy. The psychiatrist may wish to come up with his own conclusory opinion (and indeed in many expert witness roles he is required to do so), but it is never sufficient for him merely to present a conclusion without supporting data. Ultimately, the clinical information which the psychiatrist is able to convey to the judge or jury should be of as great or greater value than the psychiatrist's opinion, particularly when that opinion involves an elusive area such as dangerousness, competency, or criminal responsibility.

What Types of Attitudes and Behaviors Make the Psychiatrist a Good Witness?

Once the psychiatrist takes the stand, his attorney will inquire as to the doctor's qualifications. Then the attorney will ask the doctor to report on the circumstances of his examination and his findings. In responding to this inquiry, the doctor should be thorough yet crisp. It is extremely important to avoid jargon. When the psychiatrist accidentally slips into using medical terms, it is wise for him to stop, correct himself, and explain the meaning of such terms. It is not easy for doctors to avoid jargon. The psychiatrist who lacks experience in communicating psychiatric concepts without using jargon should rehearse his testimony with his attorney until he has some confidence in his ability to communicate in ordinary language.

The expert witness who is committed to an adversarial position is sometimes tempted to exaggerate his expertise. This is always unwise. The psychiatrist should present himself as confident but modest. He should never hesitate to admit ignorance and be willing to say "I don't know." He should be quite willing to "sit on the fence" when he is uncertain and to acknowledge that a different set of facts or new data might cause him to change his opinion. The simplest way of capturing the best quality the psychiatrist should present to the court is that he should, whatever the situation, stick to telling only the unblemished truth. It is not unheard of for psychiatrists to exaggerate or to tell "white lies" when they become too firmly identified with the advocate position. This is a serious matter, and if dishonesty is detected the psychiatrist can be charged and convicted of perjury. The crime of perjury is a felony and a conviction can have devastating consequences for the overly eager witness.

In some trials the psychiatrist will be asked a hypothetical question which is an effort to solicit an expert opinion based on the presentation of certain alleged facts. The doctor is asked "assuming facts A, B, C, etc., to be the case, do you have an opinion?" Usually the expert will have an opinion. Upon cross-examination, however, the opposing attorney may ask if the psychiatrist's opinion would be modified if some of the facts were changed. In this instance the psychiatrist should feel perfectly free to acknowledge that he would have a different opinion with different factual material if this is actually the case.

What Should the Expert Witness Expect in the Process of Cross-Examination?

The function of cross-examination is to explore and impair, perhaps even destroy, the confidence of the judge or jury in the validity of the psychiatrist's opinion. This can be done in the following ways:

First, efforts may be made to cast doubts on the psychiatrist's credentials. Relatively inexperienced psychiatrists who are not board certified are clearly at a disadvantage in this situation. There is nothing they can do about this other than showing their ability through the quality of their testimony.

Second, efforts might be made to indicate that the psychiatrist's testimony is suspect because he is a "professional witness." The psychiatrist will be asked if he has testified in similar cases and inquiries will be made as to the regularity of his participation in similar cases. It is presumed that such questioning will indicate that the psychiatrist is more businesslike than idealistic, but it is hard to see how such a view of the psychiatrist should diminish his credibility. Sometimes the opposing attorney will try to question the psychiatric witness's credibility by pointing out that he is receiving a large amount of money for testifying. The psychiatrist should have no hesitation in acknowledging his fee. At the same time, he should explain that he is not simply being paid for testifying, but that rather he is being paid for his time.

Third, efforts are made to weaken the psychiatrist's testimony by attacking the factual basis of his opinion. Here the psychiatrist is protected if his examination has been extremely thorough.

Fourth, efforts may be made to question the inferences the psychiatrist has drawn from his data. Here, of course, it takes an extremely knowledgeable cross-examiner to impair the psychiatrist's opinion. Many of the younger, more knowledgeable attorneys, however, have a powerful sense of the theoretical nature of so many psychiatric inferences. Many are capable of exposing those instances in which the psychiatrist's inferences are tenuous and based on fragmentary data. Again the psychiatrist should be quite modest and humble in admitting the limitations of his expertise, should be willing to have the basis of his inferences questioned, and should not be upset when the cross-examiner points out that there are alternative explanations.

Fifth, efforts may be made to force the psychiatrist to clarify his terms and the basis of his conclusions. The psychiatric witness should be able to define any term that is used in his testimony and should clarify its exact meaning. If the psychiatrist testifies in conclusory terms without adequately stating the basis of his opinion, he of course leaves himself open to attack by a skillful cross-examiner. Conclusory testimony not buttressed by data is not only of little value to the court but may be the basis for totally discrediting the doctor's opinion.

Sixth, efforts may be made to determine if the psychiatric witness has a proper understanding of the rule of law under which he is testifying. A psychiatrist may present erroneous testimony if he is not familiar with rules which apply in a particular case and it is the task of the cross-examiner to bring this out.

Many psychiatrists tend to get upset with cross-examination and feel that it is an affront to their dignity and status. Such fear usually represents insecurity or pomposity on the part of the psychiatrist. Once again, if the psychiatrist does not become too committed to an adversarial role, he can hardly be harmed by cross-examination. It is not he who is on trial but the client. It is not he who is being attacked, only his opinion. Actually, many forensic psychiatrists, myself included, often find it a distinct pleasure to be cross-examined by a competent attorney. (And conversely, it is something of a "letdown" when the cross-examiner does a poor job.) In the process, the expert witness can learn a great deal about areas he has not considered and about alternative ways of viewing the problem. At its best, the process of cross-examination can be an exhilarating and enlightening experience for the psychiatrist. It is also reassuring to recall that much of the damage done to the psychiatrist's testimony under cross-examination can be repaired on redirect examination when his own attorney has the opportunity to examine him again and once again to clarify the strong points in his testimony.

In spite of all the reassurances that have been offered in this brief guide to the expert witness role, there will still be many psychiatrists who will find the process of testifying in court to be so terrifying as to be repugnant. It is probably true that doctors who do not enjoy competition, who do not respond well to having their opinions attacked, who have trouble responding quickly in verbal argument, and who do not have just a "touch of the ham" about them, will be wise to avoid the expert witness role. Participation in legal proceedings as an expert witness should be an enjoyable experience, both from an intellectual and emotional standpoint. If it becomes a source of agony, dread, or depression, it should be avoided.

How Much Training Does the Psychiatrist Need to Be an Expert Witness?

Some psychiatrists believe that expert witnesses need specialized training. They recommend that the future expert spend one or preferably two years studying legal issues and aspects of psychiatry that are specifically related to the law. This group has formed a new board of forensic psychiatry which certifies those who have pursued their education in this area as experts.[3]

Other psychiatrists believe that all well-trained psychiatrists should be capable of testifying as experts if they are called upon and are willing to do so.[4] These physicians argue that any competent psychiatrist should have the skills to evaluate the patient involved in litigation, to

[3]P. E. Dietz, "Forensic and Non-Forensic Psychiatrists: An Empirical Comparison," *Bulletin of the American Academy of Psychiatry and the Law 6*, no. 1 (1978): 13–22.
[4]G. L. Usdin, "Psychiatric Participation in Court," *Psychiatric Annals 7*, no. 6 (1977): 43.

learn about the legal issues involved in a specific case, and to direct their testimony toward those issues. The effectiveness of the expert, according to this group, is dependent on his psychiatric skills rather than his knowledge of legal issues or familiarity with the courtroom.

My own sympathies are primarily with the latter group. Any well-trained psychiatrist who is willing to be an expert witness and who enjoys the process is quite capable of mastering the small amount of legal information he needs to be an effective witness. In fact, the occasional witness may be just as effective or more effective than the board-certified forensic psychiatrist. Ultimately, it is the quality of psychiatric evaluation rather than knowledge of legal issues which makes for effective testimony.

To What Extent Does Participation in Expert Witness Roles Have Political Consequences?

Almost any psychiatric intervention has political consequences and courtroom psychiatry is no exception. Some trials involving psychiatric testimony lead to changes in the law. Some psychiatrists, including myself, have volunteered our services in civil rights cases in order to advance a social position. When the psychiatrist assists in *amicus curiae* briefs he in effect becomes a lobbyist for his own organization and for certain ideological positions.

On the other hand, psychiatric testimony can also help to stabilize the status quo. Nowhere has this accusation been made more stridently than with respect to psychiatric participation in the area of civil commitment. Here we are accused of helping to negate social protest and social variation by labeling deviancy as illness and depriving the person who is "different" of freedom.[5] Although with occasional exceptions this accusation represents a distortion, similar but more muted accusations about other aspects of forensic psychiatry have some cogency. Psychiatric participation in the insanity trial and the incompetency proceeding does help to strengthen our current system of correctional justice. Psychiatric participation in disputes over wills, contracts, and child custody often favors legal decisions which reflect the prevailing morality of the society and which penalize the litigant whose morality or behavior is at variance with society. In both criminal and civil trials in which psychiatrists participate there is always the risk that the courts and society will avoid examining moral problems in sufficient detail because they are satisfied that medical expertise has already provided explanations.

[5]N. Kittrie, *The Right to Be Different* (Baltimore; Johns Hopkins University Press, 1971).

Many cases in which psychiatrists testify do raise serious moral issues. If these are not examined by society, the likelihood of social change is diminished and the status quo is strengthened.

The sensitive psychiatrist appreciates that his participation as an expert will, in addition to affecting the litigants, have at least some influence on the society as a whole. The influence on society may be negligible, but it exists and it does not escape the attention of our critics. Awareness of political and ethical issues makes the psychiatrist a better clinician and a better witness.

It is likely that ethical and political issues play at least some role in the psychiatrist's selection of cases in which he will testify. The psychiatrist does not or should not simply provide his services to whichever client will pay him. Rather, he must have some belief in the case of the client for whom he testifies. The psychiatrist may also want to participate primarily in cases which may favor slight social changes in directions he favors. As one who has only a limited amount of time to devote to courtroom work, for example, I testify primarily in civil rights cases, civil commitment proceedings, psychic injury cases, or in malpractice suits which provide an opportunity to establish ethical standards of practice. Other psychiatrists probably have quite different patterns of case selection which, like mine, are likely to be partly determined by their ideology.

11

The Psychiatric Witness and the Insanity Defense

When a layperson pictures a psychiatrist in court, the most likely image is that of a doctor testifying about the nature of an offender's mental condition at the time of committing a crime. The legal question of what should be done with a person who commits an offense when he is mentally ill and seemingly out of control of his actions has perplexed and fascinated the civilized world for centuries. Over two thousand years ago the Greeks and Romans accepted the notion that an individual must have free choice if he is to be held morally and legally responsible for his actions. In both ancient cultures, individuals who were mentally ill were sometimes viewed as deprived of free choice and, therefore, unable to have the requisite mental state (guilty mind or criminal intent) to be held responsible for criminal behavior. In Anglo-American law, proof of a mental element of criminal intent is required before a person can be found guilty of a crime, and the absence of such intent has been used to exculpate certain mentally ill people since the eleventh century. Historians are fond of commenting on the manner in which treatises on the insanity defense are characterized by a consistent focusing on the same issues regardless of the century in which they are written.[1] Apparently the insanity defense has captured the imagination of legal scholars, the public, and doctors in identical ways at different times throughout history.

One view of the insanity defense is that it provides a mechanism by which an individual can be excused from taking responsibility for committing an antisocial act. Psychiatrists as physicians are familiar with the role of providing excuses which allow disabled people to avoid cer-

[1] J. M. Quen, "Anglo-American Criminal Insanity: An Historical Perspective," *Bulletin of the American Academy of Psychiatry and the Law 2*, no. 2, (1974): 115–23.

tain obligations. Physically disabled individuals, for example, are not held to the same standards of conduct in our society as others. They may receive income without working and they are usually excused from military service. Mental illness can also be an excusing condition for fulfilling contractual obligations and for performing military service. Until recent years, mental illness was the major reason for allowing pregnant women to receive therapeutic abortions and thereby to be excused from childbearing. Perhaps because psychiatrists are so familiar with the excuse-giving role they have tended to accept the relevance of the insanity defense and to view their participation in such litigation as natural and proper.[2] Medical testimony in the insanity trial has been available to the courts and welcomed by them since the eighteenth century.

How Frequently Is the Insanity Defense Raised and How Frequently Does It Result in Acquittal?

The precise answer to both questions depends on the locality, but in general the insanity defense is rarely invoked and is rarely successful. The majority of insanity pleas are lost; in New York in the decade of the 1960s, there were only eleven successful insanity defenses. In the state of North Carolina there have thus far been only two acquittals in the 1970s. Even in the District of Columbia during the years when the *Durham* decision (a ruling which allowed for exceptionally broad interpretations of insanity) was in effect, acquittals by reason of insanity never rose above 5% of all criminal cases terminated. (One reason the insanity defense may be invoked in a district where there is little likelihood of its being successful is to find a way of bringing psychiatric testimony into the trial. Such testimony might not excuse, but it might mitigate the harshness of punishment imposed. It is unlikely, however, that psychiatric input during the determination of guilt or innocence has a significant effect on sentencing if the defendant is eventually found guilty.)

If the Use of the Insanity Defense Has so Little Impact, in Terms of Numbers, on Offenders or the Criminal Justice System, Why Has the Defense Received so Much Attention?

Legal scholars have pondered the reason for the fascination so many individuals have had with this issue for so long. One source of

[2]S. L. Halleck, "The Power of the Psychiatric Excuse," *Marquette Law Review* 52, no. 2 (1970).

fascination is that the insanity defense calls our attention to critical moral issues involving the assignment of blame, responsibility, and punishment. When the issue of insanity is interjected, blame, responsibility, and punishment must be considered in the light of the possibility that there are mental conditions which compromise an individual's free will. This usually leads into a free will versus determinism debate and challenges society to try to define the conditions under which free will may or may not exist. Arguments that people do not always exert free will may threaten the basis of our legal system, our theological beliefs, and our basic assumptions about the nature of man. Many fear that if the concept of determinism were applied too broadly in dealing with issues of blame, responsibility, and punishment, the basic rules of conduct which hold our society together would be unenforceable. Most intellectuals keep a close watch on the insanity defense, and though they take various stances on how broad or narrow the range of excusability should be, they realize that too much broadening can have profound moral and political consequences for the entire society.

What are the Moral and Legal Justifications of the Insanity Defense?

Legal scholars are unclear as to how to answer this question. One obvious formulation is that an insane person cannot be held morally responsible for committing an illegal act because his disease deprives him of choice or free will. Sometimes, the insanity defense is linked to the mental element of a crime or the issue of criminal intent. To be guilty of a crime a subject must not only have committed an illegal act (*actus reas*) but must also be proven to have possessed a mental state which is a requisite element of that crime. (*mens rea,* or a "guilty mind"). The insane person can be viewed as lacking the capacity to have the mental element required in defining a crime, and, therefore, as not blameworthy or punishable. Whether the insanity defense is technically a *mens rea* issue is, however, debatable. Another argument which is often used to justify the insanity defense is that the mentally ill person would probably not be deterred by the threat of punishment nor would his punishment serve as a proper example of an individual whose punishment would deter others from committing a similar crime. If an individual is so disturbed as not to be influenced by the deterrent function of the criminal law, the case for excusing him from the punitive sanctions of the law is strengthened.[3]

[3]A. Stone, *Mental Health and Law: A System in Transition* (Rockville, Md.: NIMH, 1975), chap. 13.

How Does the Use of the Insanity Defense Vary with Changing Social Conditions?

Throughout history the finding that a given defendant is not guilty by reason of insanity has not meant that he has been set free. The usual consequence of such acquittal is that the defendant, although held not to be responsible for the crime, is nevertheless restrained in an institutional setting, usually a hospital for the criminally insane. This has been justified traditionally by the assumption that the person probably has committed the physical act of the crime, is likely to do it again, and is a danger to society. In effect, the acquitted patient has often faced punitive sanctions which potentially are as aversive as those imposed on the guilty. Conditions of everyday life in hospitals for the criminally insane are often little better than those in prisons. In addition, defendants sent to an institution for the criminally insane after being found not guilty by reason of insanity are not offered the certainty of a fixed maximum period of confinement. In past years they faced the possibility of spending as long or longer in custodial care as they would have if convicted of the original charge. More recently this risk has diminished, but it has not entirely disappeared. For these reasons the insanity defense has been used primarily in situations where the crime for which the offender is accused is a serious one which is likely to result in a long sentence or execution once guilt is determined. So many insanity defenses in past years have involved capital crimes that some legal scholars have argued that the insanity defense arose primarily out of an effort to shield highly disturbed individuals from the death penalty.[4]

The probability of a defendant's invoking the insanity defense will be influenced by existing sentencing practices and by existing regulations regarding the disposition of those found not guilty by reason of insanity. Where the probable sentence for a given crime is light, fewer individuals charged with that crime will plead insanity. When penalties are severe, the number of insanity pleas will increase. If there is little probability of avoiding prolonged custodial care following an acquittal by reason of insanity, fewer individuals will invoke the insanity defense. If there is considerable likelihood that an individual found not guilty by reason of insanity can gain relatively quick release or complete freedom, the use of the insanity defense will increase.

A brief review of current trends in our criminal justice and mental health systems would suggest that conditions are ripe for a rapid expansion of use of the insanity defense. Many states are currently imposing

[4]A. L. Halpern, "The Insanity Defense: A Juridicial Anachronism," *Psychiatric Annals 7*, no. 8 (1977).

stiff penalties for a large variety of crimes. Fixed sentencing which is now fashionable provides the offender with even less hope of a light penalty. In addition, efforts to reinstate the death penalty have gained powerful impetus within the last decade and are supported by the majority of the public. As the criminal justice system becomes more punitive we can anticipate that more and more defendants will invoke the insanity defense to avoid harsh retribution. At the same time the rights of patients found not guilty by reason of insanity have been expanded. Some recent court rulings suggest that it will become increasingly difficult to restrain these individuals for long periods in institutions for the criminally insane. Our courts are accepting that once the defendant has been found not guilty and hospitalized, he is entitled to be treated and to be released when cured. For that matter the courts may be ready to approve outright release of many found not guilty by reason of insanity. After all, the defendant is quite likely to be reasonably sound from a mental standpoint at the time of acquittal since the very fact that he was able to stand trial means that he was considered to be competent and legally sane at the moment the trial ended.

In 1968 a federal court of appeals argued that a hearing was necessary before a person found not guilty by reason of insanity could be committed to a mental hospital.[5] In a 1972 ruling on the indefinite compulsory detention of individuals found incompetent to stand trial, the Supreme Court has put substantial limitations on how long these individuals can be restrained in a hospital for the criminally insane.[6] A 1975 New Jersey Supreme Court ruling held that the commitment and treatment of persons found not guilty by reason of insanity must be substantially similar to the commitment and treatment of civilly committed persons. If the defendant is not found to be still mentally ill and dangerous at the time of acquittal, he is entitled to release.[7] As we begin to see more defendants gaining freedom as a result of a successful insanity defense we should anticipate a marked increase in its use.

Those involved in the administration of criminal justice as well as the public are aware of these trends. They have recently shown greater concern with the possibility that the increased use of the insanity defense will allow too many offenders to escape justice. We are beginning to see more arguments for abolition of the insanity defense based on the concern that it allows offenders to "beat the rap." The fear that the insanity defense will allow some offenders to escape justice may become a force toward diminishing its successful use. Judges and juries are

---

[5]Bolton v. Harris, 395 F. 642 (D.C. Cir. 1968).
[6]Jackson v. Indiana, 406 U.S. 715, 737 (1972).
[7]State v. Krol, 68 N.J. 236, 344 A.2d 289 (1975).

influenced by knowledge that the acquitted offender might go free. As long as they believe the supposedly dangerous offender will be institutionalized anyway, they may not be too troubled when reaching a verdict of not guilty by reason of insanity. But to the extent that acquittal by reason of insanity means complete freedom for the defendant, such a verdict may become much more difficult to achieve.

There may be still other developments in the legal and mental health field which are influencing the frequency of use of the insanity defense. As crime rates and rates of apprehension of offenders have increased, the criminal justice system has experienced increasing difficulty in disposing of offenders by imprisonment. Traditionally that system has diverted a large number of offenders or suspected offenders away from prisons through such devices as probation, financial penalties, work release, or funneling them into a different system of control. The latter device is commonly utilized and many suspected offenders are sent directly to mental health systems. Police officers, who have a great deal of discretionary power, when arresting an individual who has just committed a deviant act can decide that he is mentally ill and bring him to a hospital rather than to jail. Judges at the time of arraignment often hold out the promise of dropping charges if the offender is willing to enter a mental hospital. And as will be pointed out in the next chapter, a large number of offenders are found incompetent to stand trial and some of them have spent large amounts of time in hospitals for the criminally insane, have never been tried, and have never gone to prison. But the mental health reform movement has made it substantially more difficult to send possible offenders to mental hospitals and keep them there. It has also spawned court decisions which limit the amount of time for which incompetent individuals can be diverted from the criminal justice system. These changes may increase the pool of mentally disturbed offenders who are brought to trial and who will seek diversion from imprisonment through the insanity defense.

What Does the Term "Insanity" Mean in the Context of the Insanity Defense, and How Is the Psychiatrist Asked to Provide Expertise in Determining Its Presence?

Insanity is a legal term, not a medical term. It refers to a legal excusing condition which has two elements; some form of mental illness and some form of incapacity which is believed to be related to that illness. In most insanity tests it is the incapacity rather than the mental illness which is the critical excusing condition. It is important for the psychiatrist to realize that the term "insanity" cannot be equated with the term "mental illness" or the term "psychosis." Many severely disturbed patients will not be found insane because they do not have the specific incapacities the court views as excusing conditions.

It is also critical that the psychiatrist be constantly aware that the question of whether the offender is sane or insane is always a judgment made by the judge or jury. One reason the term "insanity" is not equated with mental illness and is not defined in medical terms is to provide the judge and jury with the opportunity to consider moral issues in ascribing responsibility and guilt.

If insanity is indeed a legal concept, its presence or absence could arguably be decided by a judge or jury without the testimony of a psychiatrist. Determining whether an individual should be justly held responsible for his criminal actions should not always require the testimony of medical experts. In theory at least, an insanity trial could be held and justly decided without the judge's or jury's hearing one word of psychiatric testimony. In the modern era, of course, this never happens. The court insists on psychiatric testimony for three purposes: first, to provide facts as to the offender's illness; second, to offer opinions as to the nature of that illness; and third, to offer opinions as to whether the patient's illness was such as to have made him legally insane at the time of the crime under the standards of insanity employed in that jurisdiction. The first two tasks are relatively straightforward and familiar to the psychiatrist. We can give facts and opinions about the mental status of offenders at the time we examine them and we can provide less valid, but still useful, opinions as to their mental status at the time they alledgedly committed a crime. The third task is more difficult and from a scientific perspective probably impossible. Translating clinical data into opinions as to how mental illness makes a person legally insane and negates his responsibility for a criminal act is a task for which a psychiatrist has no training, no science, and no theories to guide him. (I will elaborate on this argument in a later part of this chapter.) Like anyone else, the psychiatrist may have moral viewpoints as to an offender's responsibility. But when he is asked whether or not an offender meets the standards of insanity, his response may be presumed to be an expert rather than a moral opinion. The courts, our society, and many psychiatrists tend to view such testimony as scientific.

There is a blurring of scientific and moralistic perspectives here. Nevertheless, the courts (with the exception of a brief period of time in which the District of Columbia Court of Appeals discouraged psychiatrists from making conclusory statements as to an offender's insanity) assume that the psychiatrist will give conclusory testimony to a moral and legal question.[8] Even if a given court did not insist on the psychiatrist's testifying in a conclusory manner, it would be extremely difficult for the psychiatrist to do otherwise. I have on a number of occasions offered to go to court in insanity cases and testify as to the nature of the offender's illness and as to how it may have influenced his criminal behavior, but have indicated that I could not make conclusory statements as to the offender's responsibility under any standard of insanity. No attorney has accepted my offer, primarily because they assume that if the opposing side employs a psychiatrist who does make a conclusory statement, that psychiatrist's testimony will carry more weight than mine and will prevail.

What Are the Various Tests or Standards That Are Used or Have Been Used to Determine Insanity?

The most important and time-honored test currently used is the *M'Naghton* test. It reads:

> Every man is to be presumed to be sane, and . . . to establish a defense on the grounds on insanity, it must be clearly proved that, at the time of the committing of the act, the party accused was laboring under a defect of reason, from disease of the mind, as not to know the nature and quality of the act he was doing; or if he did know it, that he did not know he was doing what was wrong.

One writer has noted that the quest for an excuse here can be phrased "I did not know what I was doing" or "I didn't know that what I did was wrong."[9]

In a number of states an irresistible impulse test may be added to the *M'Naghton* test. The federal standard which contains an irresistible impulse clause reads as follows: "[The accused is to be classified as insane if] though conscious of [the nature of the act] and able to distinguish right from wrong . . . yet his will, by which I mean the governing power of his mind has been otherwise involuntarily so completely destroyed that his actions are not subject to it, but are beyond his control."[10]

The excusing rationale here can be paraphrased as "I couldn't help it."

The American Law Institute (ALI) test, which is gaining increasing

---

[8]R. J. Bonnie, "Commentary: Criminal Responsibility," in *Diagnosis and Debate,* edited by R. J. Bonnie. (New York: Insight Communications, 1977), pp. 97–98.
[9]A. Brooks, *Law, Psychiatry and the Mental Health System* (Boston: Little, Brown 1973).
[10]Brooks, *Law, Psychiatry and the Mental Health System.*

popularity in many states and which has just recently been adopted by California, reads:

> 1. A person is not responsible for criminal conduct if, at the time of such conduct as a result of mental disease or defect, he lacks substantial capacity either to appreciate the criminality of his conduct or to conform his conduct to the requirements of the law.
>
> 2. As noted in the article, the terms "mental disease or defect" do not include an abnormality manifested only by repeated criminal or otherwise antisocial conduct.[11]

The ALI test includes elements of "I didn't know what I was doing or that it was wrong" and "I couldn't help it."

The *Durham* test, which is no longer used but which is of considerable historical interest to legal scholars and psychiatrists, reads:

> An accused is not criminally responsible if his unlawful act was the product of mental disease or mental defect.... we use "disease" in the sense of a condition which is considered capable of either improving or deteriorating. We use "defect" in the sense of a condition which is not considered capable of either improving or deteriorating and which may be either congenital, or the result of injury, or the residual effect of a physical or mental disease.[12]

The excusing phrase behind *Durham* might be paraphrased "I couldn't help doing it because I was mentally ill."

The major tests currently in use in the United States are the *M'Naghton* and the ALI. Each has its critics and proponents. It is generally argued that the *M'Naghton* test puts major emphasis on cognitive disabilities and the ALI test on affective disabilities. Generally, the ALI test is viewed as broadening the range of excusability and as more likely to accommodate psychiatric testimony.[13]

Psychiatrists initially hailed the *Durham* test as one which would free them to testify scientifically and which might excuse a greater number of mentally ill offenders. While *Durham* did result in an increase in the frequency of acquittals by reason of insanity in the District of Columbia, it is questionable whether conclusory statements that a crime is a product of a mental illness can be considered scientific. (Mental illness may be a necessary cause of a criminal act, but it is difficult to see how it could be a sufficient cause. The term "product" implies sufficient causality.) Jurists were greatly troubled by the vagueness of *Durham*. It was felt that the test gave too much discretion to the psychiatrists who usually failed to meet the challenge of providing the comprehensive

[11]Brooks, *Law, Psychiatry and the Mental Health System.*
[12]Halleck, "The Power of the Psychiatric Excuse."
[13]Y. Rennie, *The Search for Criminal Man* (Lexington, Mass.: D. C. Heath, 1978), chap. 24.

testimony some courts wanted but instead made conclusory statements which were inadequately explained to the judge or jury. At any rate, the *Durham* test was repeatedly modified and eventually abandoned as unworkable.[14]

The psychiatrist who testifies in an insanity case must know which test is being employed. He must try to provide testimony which will enable the judge or jury to determine whether insanity, as defined by the criteria of that test, is either present or absent. It is important to note that both of the currently employed tests use phrases such as "knowing the nature and quality of the act," "appreciating the criminality of one's conduct," or "inability to conform his conduct to the requirements of law." The psychiatrist is asked to make definitive responses to questions which employ these phrases. Again, many psychiatrists, including myself, do not believe that we have any skills which enable us to give scientific responses to such questions. In my own experience I have never known an offender who did not know the nature and quality of his act or appreciate the criminality of his conduct. Nor do I know of any facts or theories which enable me to judge whether an offender has sufficient control of his impulses to obey the law. Any responses I make to these questions would ultimately be contaminated by my moral views as to whether I felt the offender was responsible and punishable. The psychiatrist, unless specifically requested not to give conclusory testimony, will under any of the current standards be asked to make a moral rather than a scientific judgment. This, in my opinion, is asking too much of the expert witness.

What Information Do Psychiatrists Actually Have Regarding the Issue of Responsibility and What Information Could Psychiatrists Supply to the Court That Might Be Helpful in Making Decisions as to an Offender's Insanity?

The theories of psychiatry and all the mental health disciplines are based on scientific determinism. We assume that behavior is determined by an individual's interaction with the environment. An individual's genetic makeup, all his previous learning experiences, and the nature of environmental experiences which impinge upon him at any given moment interact in an extremely complex manner to elicit any given behavior. Whereas we acknowledge that we may never be able to define all the elements that determine behavior, we nevertheless believe that such

[14]L. E. Becker, "Durham Revisited," *Psychiatric Annals 3,* no. 8 (1973).

elements exist. Some observers have wondered how a profession completely committed to a deterministic theory of the causes of behavior can possibly contribute to the problems of a legal system which must be concerned with the morality of behavior and must assume that people have free will to choose to behave in either a blameworthy or socially acceptable manner. It has been argued that these two philosophical views of man can never be reconciled.[15] I believe, however, that there is a way of viewing this problem which provides some insights into ways of integrating these opposing views.

Although psychiatrists are determinists, their interaction with patients suggests that they assume the existence of free will. Even though we view behavior as determined, we regularly admonish our patients to take responsibility for their actions. Indeed, psychotherapy is not likely to be successful unless the patient learns to hold himself accountable for all his thoughts and actions, and even for his unconscious motivations. Questions such as "What do you want to do about that?" or "What did you do to create this situation?" are routinely asked of patients in most forms of psychotherapy. We teach patients to formulate their motivations in terms of wishes or wants instead of needs. When the patient seems to be taking responsibility for his thoughts and actions, we reinforce him. When the patient eschews responsibility, we fail to provide reinforcement or we may respond to him in a critical manner. Even when we venture away from the psychotherapeutic process and offer advice on issues such as childrearing, we sound like staunch believers in free will. Psychiatrists, like all other behavioral scientists, recommend childrearing methods in which children are taught to behave responsibly. We advocate teaching children to feel good about themselves when they "choose" to behave in a correct way and to feel bad about themselves when they "choose" to behave badly. How can the apparent contradiction between our theoretical commitment to determinism and our practical use of therapeutic and educational methods which assume the patient's free will or responsibility be reconciled?

The most parsimonious explanation is that psychiatrists use the concept of responsibility to manipulate behavior. A demand that a person behave responsibly, and that rewards will follow if he complies and that punishments will follow if he does not, is in effect a technique for shaping or determining behavior. The patient's belief that he can choose to behave well or badly increases his susceptibility to both internal and external reinforcements. Stated differently, the concept of responsibility is simply an idea, an expectation, a viewpoint (or possibly a myth) that is inculcated into people in order to increase the probabilities that they will

---

[15]Stone, *Mental Health and Law*, p. 227.

behave in a certain way. In an apparently paradoxical manner, a person's belief in his own free will is only one more factor which determines his behavior.

It is easy to generalize from this model and argue that society also manipulates behavior and must demand responsible behavior if it is to function efficiently. We train people from an early age to believe that they have considerable control over their destiny. Children learn that they will be rewarded for good behavior and punished for bad behavior. They also learn to reward and punish themselves for good or bad behavior. Again, although it is impossible to prove that free will does or does not exist, the automatic assumption of its existence helps to shape a law-abiding society. Just as the competent psychiatrist manipulates the concept of responsibility to shape his patients' behavior in a "healthy" manner, the efficient and just society manipulates the concept of responsibility to induce good citizenship and law-abiding behavior.

The above model may help clarify the futility of psychiatrists' trying to testify scientifically according to current standards for determining insanity. The legal system must impose blame in order to shape a law-abiding society. But the psychiatrist knows (or should know) that blame or responsibility cannot be defined or measured scientifically. We can only define and measure the manner in which sanctions and learning that demand responsibility influence behavior. The model, however, does suggest ways in which scientific testimony could help the courts in making moral decisions.

Psychiatrists do have some scientific ability to determine an offender's capacity to evaluate the benefits and risks of a given criminal act. A variety of factors outside an individual's control may alter his capacity to make accurate and adaptive risk–benefit evaluations with regard to criminal actions.

Distorted early learning experiences and maternal deprivation may so influence an individual that he comes to value unrealistically the benefits of certain actions such as violence. A variety of mental illnesses may also distort an individual's perception of the benefits of a criminal act and may certainly alter his capacity to perceive the risks of that act. Patients who cannot evaluate risks may not be deterrable by the threat of punishment. Nor is punishing them likely to set a meaningful example that would deter others. Society may not want to hold these individuals fully responsible for criminal acts and may not wish to punish them too harshly.

A comprehensive listing of all the factors which interfere with an individual's capacity to make adaptive risk–benefit evaluations of criminal actions would include many sociological as well as psychobiological factors. In fairness, sociological as well as psychiatric testimony might be considered in determining the desirability or degree of punishment. A rational view of how an individual's behavior is determined might open the courts to considering a wide variety of excusing or mitigating circumstances. It should be clear, however, that viewing sociological variables as excusing conditions would create serious problems for our criminal justice system. Most apprehended and indicted defendants are likely to have experienced considerable economic deprivation and social stress. Our courts would not be receptive to the idea of looking for excusing conditions in the majority of criminal proceedings, particularly when they believe that "sociological criminals," unlike insane criminals, are deterable by punishment.

There is little likelihood that there will be significant changes in tests for insanity or in the use of psychiatric testimony in the near future. Psychiatrists will continue to be asked to translate their clinical observations into moral judgments as to the responsibility and guilt of offenders who plead insanity. There are, of course, many psychiatrists who believe that they can determine when mental illness so affects an individual as to render him incapable of knowing what he is doing, knowing that it is wrong, or being unable to control his actions. These are the doctors who are most likely to testify in insanity cases. There are other psychiatrists, like myself, who believe that it is impossible to make these determinations on a scientific basis and that the psychiatrist's responses will be largely determined by his personal morality. These psychiatrists avoid the expert witness role in criminal insanity trials. The psychiatrist who does testify must be aware that he risks a certain amount of disapproval from the public and his colleagues. In highly publicized and controversial cases, psychiatrists for the defendant and for the prosecution will come up with quite similar descriptions of the defendant's mental illness and its causes. Then one psychiatrist will say that the defendant should be excused under the standards of the *M'Naghton* or ALI tests and the other will say that he should not. It is at this point that the "battle of experts" makes psychiatry look disturbingly unscientific. My contention is that there is no way in which psychiatrists can look or be scientific when they are debating moral concepts such as legal insanity.

If the Psychiatrist Decides to Be a Witness in an Insanity Trial, What Are Some of the Issues He Must Anticipate?

The psychiatrist may become involved in the insanity trial as a defense witness, as a prosecution witness, or as an impartial witness appointed by the court. In each instance he must examine the defendant after the crime has actually occurred and will have no firsthand information as to the patient's mental status at the time of the crime. The patient's current mental status may tell the psychiatrist very little about what the patient was like many weeks or months earlier. By the time the psychiatrist conducts his examination, the defendant may already have been found competent to stand trial and the acute condition which was alleged to have been present at the time of the crime may have long since disappeared. Or the patient may have developed new symptoms as a result of the stresses of arrest, indictment, and being jailed. The task of trying to figure out what a person's mental status was months or years ago is complicated further when the patient's recollection of events is not good or if the patient is motivated to distort facts. Often the psychiatrist must rely heavily on information obtained from others. It is useful to examine the police report of the crime, to interview or read the statements of people who were in close contact with the patient preceding, during, or following the crime, and to obtain objective information as to the patient's past history from relatives.

Participation in the insanity defense requires that the psychiatrist be extremely well prepared and thorough. An hour or two of interviewing simply will not suffice. To be a good witness the psychiatrist must review every report available about the defendant, must interview all significant individuals who are available, and must spend many hours with the defendant reconstructing the details of his illness, the criminal event, and how the illness and crime might be related. On the witness stand, it is advisable to anticipate vigorous cross-examination. The psychiatrist working for the defendant will have an especially difficult time trying to make a case for the defendant's insanity at the time of the crime since at the time of the trial the defendant, who must be competent to stand trial, is likely to look quite normal.

What Is the Concept of "Partial Responsibility" and How Does It Relate to Psychiatric Testimony?

The term "partial responsibility" refers to a legal means of reducing the severity of the crime with which the defendant is charged or the severity of sentencing on the basis of testimony as to the defendant's mental state. In several states the mental state of the offender is considered in formulating charges and in setting punishment. A defendant who is intoxicated at the time he commits an offense may, for example, be charged with a less serious crime. In the state of California under the so-called *Wells–Gorshen* doctrine, testimony as to the patient's personality and emotional state can be introduced to show that the offender did not have the capacity to form the specific state of mind which is an essential element of the offense for which he is charged.[16] If an offender, for example, does not have the required state of mind to be charged with first-degree murder, a lesser charge may be made.

There are no consistent standards or formulae to which the psychiatrist must testify in determination of the offender's capacity to form a specific intent. The psychiatrist can describe the patient's illness and provide opinions as to how the patient's emotional state may have influenced the crime. The court makes the legal decision as to whether the defendant possessed the requisite mental element.

The use of psychiatric testimony is likely to be increasingly utilized in the process of sentencing. Under currently popular determinate sentencing laws instituted in several states, the judge must impose a relatively fixed sentence but mitigating or aggravating circumstances may influence its length. Conceivably, the psychiatrist could be called in to document aspects of the offender's mental condition which would lead to a harsher sentence, but as a rule the psychiatrist will testify as to mitigating circumstances such as the existence of an emotional illness at the time of the crime which might justify a lesser sentence.

In the state of North Carolina, offenders convicted of capital crimes are entitled to a hearing at which mitigating circumstances can be considered before the death penalty is imposed. One mitigating circumstance is the presence of an emotional disorder which may have been a factor in causing the crime. Here the psychiatrist does not have to testify as to any specific standards but can simply describe in a relatively scientific manner how the patient's emotional state influenced his capacity to evaluate the risks and benefits of a particular crime. The introduction of testimony regarding emotional disorders as mitigating circumstances raises the possibility that sociological, as well as psychological or biological factors, might be viewed as excusing conditions. The psychiatrist may wish to invoke sociological data in developing a holistic picture of the causation of a given crime, but as noted, the courts will be wary of viewing social deprivation or oppression as a mitigating circumstance.

What Are Some of the Arguments for and against Retaining the Insanity Defense?

In the last two decades, there has been continuous debate as to whether the insanity defense is useful or detrimental to society. Most

---

[16]People v. Wells, 202 P.2d 53, 62–63 (Cal. 1949), *Cert. denied* 337 U.S. 919; People v. Gorshen, 336 P.2d 492, 503 (Cal. 1959).

psychiatrists do not as a rule become involved in this debate, but it may be useful for the practicing psychiatrist at least to be aware of the arguments of each side. Those who favor retention of the insanity defense argue that it is morally sound not to punish those who are sick, who lack the capacity to make reasonable choices, and who are not deterrable.[17] They also point out that if the insanity defense is truly based on the concept of *mens rea* or guilty mind, it would probably be unconstitutional to outlaw the insanity defense since there would then be no opportunity for the defendant to prove that that intent was not present.[18] Other proponents have argued that the insanity defense helps to stabilize the entire criminal justice system.[19] If only a few individuals who are extremely disturbed are found not guilty by reason of insanity, it can be assumed that the great majority who are found guilty must be responsible individuals who are justly punished.[20] Finally, it has been argued that the insanity defense allows for diversion of a certain number of criminal offenders and is in that sense a "safety valve" for an already overburdened and overcrowded correctional system.[21]

Those who wish to abolish the insanity defense point out that its use results in expensive trials and that it accomplishes little insofar as it usually results in offenders' being institutionalized anyway.[22] An extremely telling argument is that the insanity defense is rarely available to the indigent defendant. As a rule, the fate of the indigent defendant is determined by the report of the court-appointed psychiatrist. It is rare for a poor person to be able to employ his own psychiatrist who might have a different opinion than the state-employed psychiatrist.[23] Some critics fear that the insanity defense allows too many offenders to escape punishment.[24] Critics of a different political persuasion fear that indeterminate commitment which follows the acquittal by reason of insanity presents too many threats to the civil rights of the defendant, who might be better off in jail.[25]

[17]S. Pollack, "The Insanity Defense as Defined by the Proposed Federal Criminal Code," *Bulletin of the American Academy of Psychiatry and the Law 4*, no. 1 (1976): 11–23.

[18]A. Goldstein, *The Insanity Defense* (New Haven, Conn.: Yale University Press, 1967).

[19]J. Monahan, "Abolish the Insanity Defense?—Not Yet," *Rutgers Law Review 26* (1973): 719.

[20]J. Hall, "Mental Disease and Criminal Responsibility: M'Naghten v. Durham," *Indiana Law Journal 33* (1958): 212–25.

[21]Bonnie, "Criminal Responsibility," p. 101.

[22]S. L. Halleck, *Psychiatry and the Dilemmas of Crime* Harper, 1967.

[23]Becker, "Durham Revisited."

[24]A. Dershowitz, "Abolishing the Insanity Defense: The Most Significant Feature of the Administration's Proposed Code—An Essay, *Criminal Law Bulletin 9* (1973): 435.

[25]T. Szasz, *Psychiatric Justice* (New York: Macmillan, 1965).

Proposals to abolish the insanity defense are accompanied by arguments for alternative means of dealing with the mentally ill offender. A common proposal is that the patient should first be found guilty of having actually performed the criminal act and that his disposition should then be determined by a treatment tribunal, including psychiatrists, who would decide what disposition, including incapacitation and treatment, are most suitable.[26] The mentally ill offender would be found guilty but would receive treatment. This model makes most sense in a correctional system which has some commitment to rehabilitation. It is becoming less relevant as our correctional system moves to determinate sentencing and puts only perfunctory emphasis on rehabilitation. It is also questionable whether total abolition of the insanity defense, as required by this model, would be constitutional. More recent arguments for abolition emphasize that such a defense is not needed because the mentally ill could still escape inordinately harsh punishment by allowing for diminution in the seriousness of charges and punishment on the basis of psychiatric testimony directed to the questions of intent and mitigating circumstances.[27] This is an arguments for relying on an expanded system of partial responsibility. Under such a system, mentally ill offenders would not be found insane but would have the opportunity to receive lesser charges and perhaps shorter sentences. This recommendation seriously troubles those who view those acquitted by reason of insanity as potentially dangerous people who should be institutionalized in one place or another. Under an expanded partial responsibility system, "dangerous" offenders might serve brief sentences and would be set free before their "dangerousness" was treated.

Finally, there are critics such as myself who are unsure as to the usefulness of the insanity defense but who have strong opinions as to the use of psychiatric testimony in these cases. Now that acquitted offenders have expanded civil rights, I would not be too troubled by the insanity defense if it were not used in a way so as to put our profession in the awkward position of having to present unscientific conclusory testimony.

Ultimately, changes in the form and use of the insanity defense will depend on future rulings by federal courts which relate to the rights of the acquitted offender and the degree to which these rulings are enforced. If it becomes apparent that more offenders are truly "getting off" by pleading insanity, we might anticipate major changes in the law which would discourage use of the defense.

[26]K. A. Menninger, *The Crime of Punishment* (New York: Viking Press, 1968).
[27]N. Morris, "Psychiatry and the Dangerous Criminal," *Southern California Law Review* 4 (1968): 514.

In What Other Ways Do Psychiatrists Contribute to "Excusing" Offenders from Punishment?

As noted previously, the judge has considerable discretion to divert offenders into the mental health system before arraignment or trial. There are many reasons why a judge may want to do this, not the least of which is to avoid the enormous expense of a possible insanity trial. Affluent patients in particular are likely to welcome diversion to private mental hospitals which often have quite comfortable accommodations and provide excellent treatment. Several years ago, in the course of running a small private hospital unit, I discovered that I had in a very brief time seen several patients who were hospitalized after being arrested for a crime. They entered my unit on the advice of their attorneys or at the request of the judge. After a brief period of treatment, the great majority of these patients either had their charges dismissed, were put on probation, or had their sentences suspended.[28] My inquiries to doctors working in other private hospitals revealed that a large proportion of their patients faced criminal charges when they entered the hospital. These doctors had experiences similar to mine and noted that the majority of patients who underwent treatment in their institutions never went to prison. In effect, it seems that there is an "underground" insanity defense for the affluent operating in this country. Anyone who commits a crime that is not too spectacular and who checks into a private mental hospital or persuades the judge to send him to one before being tried improves his chances of avoiding incarceration. No data are available on the number of cases currently diverted to this system, but it may well be that more offenders are avoiding imprisonment through the "underground" psychiatric excuse-giving mechanism than through acquittal by reason of insanity.

[28]S. L. Halleck, "A Troubled View of Current Trends in Forensic Psychiatry," *Journal of Psychiatry and Law*, Summer 1974, pp. 135–57.

12

Competency to Stand Trial

While the insanity defense has preoccupied attorneys, psychiatrists, and other scholars, the issue of incompetency to stand trial is actually of greater significance insofar as it affects many more individuals and raises just as many moral problems. More than a hundred times as many defendants are found incompetent to stand trial (and are sent to institutions for the criminally insane without having been convicted) than are acquitted on grounds of insanity.[1] The incompetency plea can be invoked by any of the participants in the criminal proceeding—the defense, the prosecution, or the court. It can be invoked at any point in the trial, and even after the defendant has already been found guilty he may still be found incompetent to be sentenced.

In recent years there has been greater appreciation on the part of those involved with the criminal justice process of the serious problems created by the incompetency plea. Some fear that it is used by offenders to "beat the rap."[2] Others fear that the incompetency plea threatens the rights of defendants by denying them their "day in court" and incarcerating them (even though they may be innocent) for an indeterminate time.[3] As will be noted later, offenders found incompetent to stand trial do lose some of the rights usually available to criminal defendants.

Psychiatrists must be concerned with the incompetency plea because the courts rely heavily on the psychiatric examination in determining incompetency to stand trial. Many more psychiatrists become involved as experts in determining whether a given individual is competent to stand trial than ever become involved in the insanity plea. Psychiatrists who work in state hospitals and hospitals for the criminally insane have a

---

[1] L. Cooke et al., "Factors Affecting Referral to Determine Competency to Stand Trial," *American Journal of Psychiatry* 130 (1973): 180.

[2] N. Steadman, *Beating a Rap* (Chicago: University of Chicago Press, 1979), chap. 1.

[3] D. B. Wexler, *Criminal Commitments and Dangerous Mental Patients: Legal Issues of Confinement, Treatment and Release* (Washington, D.C.: U.S. Government Printing Office, 1976).

special interest in the incompetency plea since they are usually given the responsibility of treating those found incompetent to stand trial.

What Are Some of the Legal Issues Involved in the Doctrine of Incompetency to Stand Trial?

According to the common law, a defendant can be so emotionally disturbed that he can be considered mentally "absent" from the trial and unable properly to assume the role of defendant. This concept is based on the doctrine of *parens patriae* and a fundamental concern for fairness. An offender, because of mental illness, may be compromised in his ability to recall events, to produce evidence, to testify in his own defense, or to confront witnesses against him. Or he may be so disturbed that he cannot project the proper demeanor to the court and maintain an effective psychological presence. The Supreme Court has consistently ruled that the conviction of a legally incompetent defendant violates his rights to due process.[4]

The argument for the incompetency plea is compelling, but in actual practice its use creates a variety of difficult problems. Once it is decided that an individual charged with a crime cannot be tried, the society must find some way of dealing with him. The alternatives are to drop the charges, to try to treat him as an outpatient until he regains his competency, or (particularly if he is felt to be dangerous) to find some way of restraining him while treatment is attempted. In practice most defendants found incompetent to stand trial have been confined to institutions, and until recently that confinement was indefinite, lasting until the defendant's competency was restored. Obviously, some defendants found incompetent will never have their competency restored and some just means must be found of dealing with them. It has become increasingly apparent to those involved in the criminal justice system that the legal and humanistic problems involved in declaring people incompetent, trying to treat them, and trying to return them to court are formidable. There are many who feel that both the offender and society are harmed by abuse of the incompetency plea and that the quest for fairness under the *parens patriae* doctrine may ultimately be more harmful than helpful.[5]

---

[4]R. Slovenko, "The Developing Law on Competency to Stand Trial," *Journal of Psychiatry and Law*, Summer 1977, pp. 165–200.
[5]A. L. Halpern, "Use and Misuse of Psychiatry in Competency Examination of Criminal Defendants," *Psychiatric Annals 5*, no. 4 (April 1975).

Is the Use of the Incompetency Plea Increasing?

The prevailing view is that the question of incompetency to stand trial is being raised with increasing frequency. More and more the question is raised by the judge. In 1966 the Supreme Court ruled that it is the judge's duty to raise the issue of competency without prompting or suggestion when there is some indication that the defendant is not competent to stand trial.[6] In a 1975 ruling, Chief Justice Burger stated that a court's failure to "resort to an adequate procedure" for determining competency when faced with substantial evidence of the defendant's mental instability violates due process of law. The Chief Justice noted that the factors to be weighed in deciding whether or not to initiate a competency inquiry include "evidence of a defendant's irrational behavior, his demeanor at the trial, and any prior medical opinion on competence to stand trial."[7] Faced with these decisions, judges wishing to avoid being overruled on appeal have tended to order competency examinations when there has been the slightest doubt about the patient's mental condition. A competency examination has become almost routine in instances where the alleged crime is in any way bizarre or spectacular.

A second reason for an increase in incompetency pleas is probably related to the recent trend toward more stringent protection of civil rights in the civil commitment process. Many patients who are now charged with minor crimes were in past years diverted from the criminal justice system and civilly committed to mental hospitals. Many of these people are no longer definable as dangerous and therefore cannot be civilly committed. When such individuals commit minor crimes these days the police may press charges and process them through the criminal justice system. (This is most likely to happen to lower socioeconomic-class offenders.) Here their history of mental illness is noted and they are ordered to be examined for competency to stand trial. It may also be true that severely disordered individuals who can no longer be hospitalized because of stringent new commitment laws now wander the streets and are more likely to become involved in activities defined as criminal than they were in past years. Conceivably, these individuals are now being charged with crimes and are also being evaluated for their competency to stand trial.

Whatever process is involved here, it does seem clear that there is a direct correlation between a tightening of laws regarding civil commit-

---

[6]Pate v. Robinson, 383 U.S. 375 (1966).
[7]Drops v. Missouri, 420 U.S. 162 (1975).

ment and an increased number of pleas of incompetency to stand trial. Offenders are being diverted from the mental health system to the criminal justice system and are then diverted back once again to a different type of mental health system (forensic hospitals or clinics for the criminally insane).

While the number of offenders ordered to be examined for competency is increasing, it is difficult to find data as to how many offenders are actually being found incompetent. As a rule one out of four of those examined is found incompetent and is usually kept in hospitals for continued treatment. The rest are returned to court relatively quickly.

Why Do the Various Actors in the Judicial Process Choose to Request Examinations for Competency?

Judges are likely to request examinations to determine the defendant's competency in the interest of fairness and to avoid being overruled on appeal. Some judges may also view the competency examination as a means of getting additional psychiatric information about the patient. It is also conceivable that the court sometimes requests examination in the hope that the patient will be found incompetent and that a long and difficult trial can be avoided. By diverting the defendant the court is spared the expense of the trial and may be able to avoid examination of very difficult moral issues. Diversion is especially convenient when the offender is assumed to be dangerous, when the case against him is weak, and when the court does not want to see him released on bail. The latter situation commonly motivates prosecutors to seek an incompetency ruling, but it may also motivate the judge.

The defense attorney may be convinced that his client is truly incompetent and should not be tried at a particular time. Or he may ask for a competency examination simply to obtain a psychiatric examination of the patient. Sometimes this information is used to make a determination as to whether a plea of not guilty by reason of insanity might later be considered. Some defense attorneys probably view the incompetency plea as a means of helping their clients "beat the rap." They hope that the patient may be civilly committed or released, or that the patient may do "easier time" in a hospital for the criminally insane than in a prison. Or the defense attorney may use the competency examination as a device to delay a trial. Sometimes a delay is accompanied by some fading of the vengeful emotions of the prosecuting witnesses and the public and may help the defendant escape such severe punishments as execution or life imprisonment.

A prosecuting attorney may ask for a competency examination to avoid having a conviction overruled on a later appeal. Or he may have a genuine wish not to convict an incompetent defendant. Too often, however, the prosecution uses the incompetency proceeding to further its own interests. A finding that the patient is incompetent usually results in postponement of the trial. The defendant is committed to a maximum-security hospital for the criminally insane until he has been restored to competency. Prosecutors have been known to invoke incompetency proceedings over the defendant's objections in order to avoid a criminal trial in situations where the state's evidence is weak. If the defendant is found incompetent, the prosecution obtains one of the results of a criminal conviction (incarceration) without giving the defendant the procedural protections of a criminal trial, including such rights as a jury trial and conviction based on proof beyond a reasonable doubt. Prosecuting attorneys also may request a determination of incompetency to ensure that the defendant will not be let out on bail. Finding a defendant incompetent to stand trial is one way prosecutors and judges can keep offenders they believe to be dangerous off the streets. It has been observed in recent years that the prosecution is more likely to request a competency examination than the defense. (The defendant is not allowed to oppose a competency examination even if it is recommended by the prosecution.) This trend should alert us to the possibility that the incompetency plea can be used primarily to exert a social control function.

What Happens to an Offender When an Examination of His Competency to Stand Trial is Requested?

In the majority of jurisdictions a request for a competency examination leads to the patient's being sent to a hospital for the criminally insane where the examination procedure may last from two to three months. During this time the patient obviously is deprived of bail. A number of commentators, both psychiatrists and attorneys, have been extremely critical of this practice.[8] It is difficult to understand why the examination of nondangerous patients cannot be conducted in an outpatient setting. It is also difficult to understand why sixty to ninety days are required to evaluate any patient, dangerous or nondangerous. Even allowing for the possibility that the observation of the patient's behavior within the hospital milieu might have some relevancy to his competency

---

[8]Group for the Advancement of Psychiatry, "Report, Misuse of Psychiatry in the Criminal Courts: Competency to Stand Trial" (New York: GAP, 1974); B. Ennis, *Prisoners of Psychiatry* (New York: Harcourt Brace Jovanovich 1974).

to behave efficiently in court (which is doubtful), it should not take more than a week or so for such observation to be made. The actual examination of the patient should not take more than a few hours.

Once the patient's examination is completed, he returns to court where the hospital report, and in some instances the report of the defendant's psychiatrist, are utilized to determine whether he is incompetent to stand trial. In the majority of instances the defendant will be found competent. (Even if the defendant had been incompetent when sent away to be examined, there is some likelihood that the two- or three-month evaluation period has been therapeutic and has restored his competency.) If a determination of incompetency is made, however, the patient is almost automatically sent back to a hospital for the criminally insane where he may remain until his competency is restored. Until 1973, when the Supreme Court ruled that there should be limits on how long incompetent offenders could be retained in hospitals for the criminally insane, incompetent defendants who had never been convicted of a crime faced lifetime incarceration. Now there are limits on how long an incompetent offender can be retained in a forensic hospital, but psychiatrists and attorneys are still troubled by the almost uniform practice of requiring persons found incompetent to be treated in institutions.[9] Many of these individuals are not dangerous to others by any criteria and could be treated safely as outpatients.

How Can the Defendant Be Harmed by Being Found Incompetent to Stand Trial?

In addition to facing lengthy institutionalization and the loss of the right to bail, the patient found incompetent to stand trial is also deprived of the advantages of plea and sentencing bargaining. As many as 95% of criminal cases in the United States are resolved not by full presentation of evidence at trial, but by a private plea-bargaining process between the prosecutor and the defense lawyer.[10] Plea bargaining is an essential part of the criminal justice system. If too large a percentage of criminal cases were actually brought to trial, the resulting expenditure of time and money would be so great that it would lead to the collapse of the entire criminal justice system. Plea bargaining gives the defendant some control over his future. If the defendant is in an incompetent "holding pattern," however, he is deprived of the opportunity to make what might be an advantageous bargain to plead guilty to a lesser sentence.

[9]A. Stone, *Mental Health and Law: A System in Transition* (Rockville, Md.: NIMH, 1975), chap. 12; Halpern, "Use and Misuse of Psychiatry."

[10]R. Slovenko, *Psychiatry and Law* (Boston: Little, Brown, 1973), p. 138.

Practices engendered by the criminal justice system's routine use of plea bargaining may also be damaging to the incompetent offender. Police and prosecutors often exaggerate or "puff" the charges in the initial postarrest stage in anticipation that the defendant will probably plead guilty to a lesser charge. In the bargaining process the agents of the state hope that by beginning with an exorbitant charge the defendant will ultimately settle for something that meets the state's idea of justice. The patient who is found incompetent to stand trial, however, cannot plea bargain. He is prevented from settling for a lesser charge that might be realistic and acceptable to him. He is then stigmatized with the original charges made against him. Because these exaggerated charges are communicated to those who confine and treat him at the hospital for the criminally insane, they are likely to view him as more dangerous than he is. He may, therefore, be subjected to aversive and unnecessary custodial restrictions.

Are Fears That Offenders Who Successfully Plead Incompetency "Beat the Rap" Justified?

A study of the disposition of thirty-five males charged with felonies who were found incompetent to stand trial in New York State between September 1, 1971, and August 31, 1972, has recently been published.[11] The "postincompetency" careers of these individuals were followed through the mental hospitals to which they were sent, back to the courts to which some were returned for continuance of their criminal processing, and finally back to their return to the streets. The author of this study concluded, "There appears little to distinguish the experiences of defendants found incompetent from those defendants who are never diverted from criminal justice procedures. It is simply doing time in a different setting. Some persons prefer that setting; others do not. The picture presented by the incompetent defendants after they return to the community is similar to that presented by strictly ex-convict groups.[12] He concludes, in effect, that these offenders did not "beat the rap." At the same time the author concedes that with the new civil rights available to the mentally disabled and with the recent Supreme Court ruling which requires that there be limits on the length of time for which a person can be restrained in a hospital for the criminally insane because of incompetency to stand trial, there is a likelihood that the incompetency approach might soon become a "better deal" for the defendant. The incompetency status might provide better living conditions and the

---

[11]Steadman, *Beating a Rap.*
[12]*Ibid.*, chap. 1.

hope of earlier release. If the defendant is "escape minded," he might also prefer to "do time" in a hospital setting where custody is usually less strict than in prison.

What Is the Legal Standard by Which Competency to Stand Trial Is Determined?

In 1960 the Supreme Court ruled unanimously that the test for competency should be "whether the defendant possesses sufficient present ability to consult with his lawyer with a reasonable degree of rational understanding and whether he has an actual as well as a factual understanding of the proceedings against him."[13] Following this ruling the majority of states have created statutes which, although varying slightly in wording, are basically equivalent to the criteria created by the Supreme Court. Either the Supreme Court's ruling or the legislation it has spawned provide the standards by which incompetency is determined.

The defendant's ability to consult with a lawyer with a reasonable degree of rational understanding and his rational as well as factual understandings of the proceedings against him are issues which may be clarified by psychiatric knowledge. But it is also true that laypeople, particularly attorneys, could probably make these judgments without the assistance of psychiatrists. One prominent forensic psychiatrist and some attorneys have questioned whether there is really need for psychiatric input into the determination of competency to stand trial.[14] They note that in most instances the psychiatrist is unlikely to know as much about the defendant's competence to stand trial as the defendant's attorney. An evaluation of whether the defendant understands the nature of the charges against him and is able to assist counsel in preparing a defense does seem to require legal knowledge. The defendant's capacity to evaluate the risks and benefits of testifying or not testifying or of pleading guilty or innocent are probably best evaluated by an attorney who knows what these risks are. Only the attorney can determine how much assistance he is going to need from the defendant in dealing with such issues as plea bargaining, direct examination of friendly witnesses, or cross-examination of adverse witnesses.

Given the standards by which incompetency is determined, there are cogent arguments for limiting the emphasis on psychiatric testimony. Nevertheless, as will shortly be noted, the psychiatrists can

[13]Dusky v. United States, 362 U.S. 402 (1960).
[14]Halpern, "Use and Misuse of Psychiatry."

provide some useful data that help the court make the ultimate legal decision. It is unlikely we will see any diminution in the demand for psychiatric testimony in this area in the near future. Raising the issue of the offender's competency will probably continue to lead to an automatic request for a psychiatric examination, and the psychiatrist's testimony will continue to exert a critical influence on the court's decision.

How Does the Psychiatrist Get Involved in the Incompetency to Stand Trial Examination?

In most jurisdictions, once a request for a competency examination has been made the offender is sent to a hospital for the criminally insane. Here the psychiatrist who is employed by that institution and who conducts the examination will be the expert witness. In some urban centers where court clinics and forensic psychiatrists are available, the court may appoint a psychiatrist who will examine a defendant who may still be in jail. In both of the above instances the psychiatrist is an impartial witness. When he functions in this role his report is likely to have a critical influence on the court's ultimate decision since his opinions are not opposed by other experts.

In more controversial cases, and particularly where the offender may happen to be affluent, both the defense and the prosecution may wish to employ their own psychiatrists and there may be a "battle of experts" as to the patient's competency. It is rare, however, for a psychiatrist to be invited to participate in an incompetency examination from an adversarial position, since the great majority of defendants are indigent and cannot afford to hire a psychiatrist.

Critics of the incompetency plea argue that the so-called neutral psychiatrist who is state employed or court appointed may not be altogether neutral, and certainly is not the patient's agent. There is clearly some inequality in justice here. An affluent defendant who may distrust or reject the opinion of the so-called impartial psychiatrist can hire his own expert. The indigent offender is denied the same opportunity.

What Errors Have Psychiatrists Commonly Made in Examining Patients for Competency to Stand Trial?

Almost every forensic textbook notes that psychiatrists tend to be ignorant as to the issues involved in the competency proceeding. Sometimes the courts show a similar lack of knowledge. As recently as the late 1960s examiners in forensic hospitals in relatively progressive states were not being asked to respond to the relevant criteria for finding incompetency. Instead the *M'Naghten* standards for determining insanity were used to determine competency.[15] Some courts did not even request the psychiatrist to respond to any criteria other than the diagnosis of psychosis. Although there is reason to hope that psychiatrists and jurists have become more knowledgeable about this area, it is still prudent to remind psychiatrists that a finding of severe mental illness, including psychotic illness, does not mean that the offender is incompetent. In fact, some psychotic patients whose emotional disorder is characterized by paranoid thinking often make good witnesses and are quite skilled in assisting in their own defense. Psychiatrists should never confuse the standards for competency with the standards of the insanity defense. The insanity defense relates to the offender's cognitive state at the time of an offense. The incompetency standard relates only to the patient's present capacity to deal with the issue of being tried. In no state are the insanity or incompetency standards even remotely identical. Psychiatrists should also be reminded that the population likely to be examined as incompetent to stand trial usually have had previous contacts with the criminal justice system, are likely to have some knowledge of the criminal law, and even in their disturbed condition may make quite adequate defendants.

Finally, psychiatrists should know that competency to perform any task, including that of being a defendant, is a quantitative rather than an absolute condition. If issues such as the offender's specific recall of each event related to an alleged crime are considered, and particularly if the psychiatrist considers an individual's ability to assist his counsel with regard to his motives and thoughts concerning the crime, then every individual probably has at least some deficits of competency and every offender may be only partially competent. No one is a perfect defendant. The psychiatrist who is assessing the defendant's competency to stand trial is only making a prediction as to that individual's capacity to be an effective defendant. There are so many variables involved in the criminal justice process that adequate prediction of this capacity will always be limited. When we have to predict how an individual might react in a variety of hypothetical situations, we can at best make probability statements. We may wish to state an opinion that a given defendant is competent or incompetent to stand trial, but it is a mistake to present simply a conclusory statement. Since we are making a prediction, it is more useful to present everything we know about an individual's mental status that leads us to make such a prediction.

---

[15]B. Ennis, "Civil Liberties Union Client 'Crazy But Competent'," *Civil Liberties in New York,* April 1969.

Careful adherence to all the above reminders should result in some diminution of the number of defendants found incompetent to stand trial. As a general rule psychiatrists find too many people incompetent. As they gain experience in forensic work, however, and familiarize themselves with the relevant legal issues, they tend to find fewer patients incompetent.

Are There Specific Criteria to Which the Psychiatrist Should Address Himself in Preparing a Report on an Offender's Competency?

Psychiatrists have attempted to devise lists of factors which should be evaluated in determining an individual's competency. Each item on the list can be weighted according to the degree of impairment the offender has in that area and an overall score can be made which is a rough mathematical expression of the individual's competency. The ultimate usefulness of such test instruments is questionable, since many different judgments must be made and since some of the items may not be relevant to the situation the defendant will ultimately face. Such lists can, however, be useful in focusing the psychiatrist's attention on relevant issues when preparing a report. The most comprehensive list has been prepared by Louis McGarry and includes the following items:

1. *Appraisal of available legal defenses:* This item calls for an assessment of the accused's awareness of his possible legal defenses, and how consistent they are with the reality of his particular circumstances.
2. *Unmanageable behaviors:* This item calls for an assessment of the appropriateness of the current motor and verbal behavior of the defendant, and the degree to which this behavior would disrupt the conduct of the trial.
3. *Quality of relating to attorneys:* This item calls for an assessment of the interpersonal capacity of the accused to relate to the average attorney. Involved are the ability to trust and to communicate relevantly.
4. *Planning of legal strategy* (including guilty pleas to lesser charges where pertinent): This item calls for an assessment of the degree to which the accused can understand, participate, and cooperate with his counsel in planning the strategy for the defense which is consistent with the reality of the circumstances.
5. *Appraisal of role* of (a) defense counsel, (b) prosecuting attorney, (c) judge, (d) jury, (e) defendant, and (f) witnesses: This set of items calls for a minimum understanding of the adversary pro-

cess by the accused. The accused should be able to identify prosecuting attorney and prosecution witnesses as foe, defense counsel as friend, the judge as neutral, and the jury as the determiners of guilt or innocence.

6. *Understanding of court procedures:* This item calls for an assessment of the degree to which the defendant understands the basic sequence of events in a trial under import for him, e.g., the different purposes of direct and cross-examination.

7. *Appreciation of charges:* This item calls for an assessment of the accused's concrete understanding of the charges against him and, to a lesser extent, the seriousness of the charges.

8. *Appreciation of range and nature of possible penalties:* This item calls for an assessment of the accused's concrete understanding and appreciation of the conditions and restrictions which could be imposed on him and their possible duration.

9. *Appraisal of likely outcome:* This item calls for an assessment of how realistically the accused perceives the likely outcome, and the degree to which impaired understanding contributes to a less adequate participation in his defense. Without adequate information on the part of the examiner regarding the facts and circumstances of the alleged offense, this item would be unratable.

10. *Capacity to disclose to attorney available pertinent facts surrounding the offense* (including the defendant's movements, timing, mental state, and actions at the time of the offense): This item calls for an assessment of the accused's capacity to give a basically consistent, rational, and relevant account of the motivational and external facts.

11. *Capacity to challenge prosecution witnesses realistically:* This item calls for an assessment of the accused's capacity to recognize distortions in prosecution testimony. Relevant factors include attentiveness and memory. In addition there is an element of initiative. If false testimony is given, the degree of activism with which the defendant will apprise his attorney of inaccuracies is important.

12. *Capacity to testify relevantly:* This item calls for an assessment of the accused's ability to testify with coherence, relevance, and independence of judgment.

13. *Self-defeating versus self-serving motivation* (legal sense): This item calls for an assessment of the accused's motivation to protect himself adequately and to utilize legal safeguards appropriately to this end. It is recognized that accused persons may be motivated to seek expiation and appropriate punishment in

their trials. Of concern here is the pathological seeking of punishment and the deliberate failure by the accused to avail himself of appropriate legal protection.[16]

While many of the judgments as to the above thirteen items can probably be made by laypersons, and may more skillfully be made by a person with legal rather than medical training, all of the items can be influenced by mental illness. The psychiatrist can be helpful to the courts by showing how the patient's illness may compromise any of the capacities listed.

How Important Is the Psychiatrist's Assessment of the Patient's Potential Disruptiveness at the Trial?

One of the thirteen items in the above list is unmanageable behavior which might disrupt the conduct of the trial. This is an important issue only if there is actually going to be a trial. As noted previously, most criminal cases are settled out of court. When unmanageable behavior is predicted psychiatrists should focus only on disruptions that may be related to mental illness. The courts have ruled that defendants whose behavior is believed to be deliberately disruptive can be tried in absentia.

Psychiatrists should also appreciate that it is extremely difficult to predict how an individual will actually behave in the courtroom. Patients who are often extremely disruptive on a psychiatric ward may suddenly become quite calm when peace officers appear to accompany them to court. When surrounded by the impressive trappings of justice symbolized by the judges' robes and by the geography and decorum of the courtroom, many patients will calm down, at least temporarily. As a general rule, psychiatrists tend to overpredict disruptiveness by assuming that hospital behavior will be generalized to courtroom behavior.

What Concerns Should the Psychiatrist Have with Regard to the Issue of Malingering When Doing an Incompetency Examination?

Although it is extremely difficult to simulate mental disease, there is no doubt that it can be done. Some offenders may feel that there are sufficient advantages to being found incompetent to stand trial to warrant an attempt at simulation. The malingerer may wish to delay the trial

---

[16]L. McGarry *et al.*, *Handbook, Competency to Stand Trial and Mental Illness* (Rockville, Md.: NIMH, 1973), pp. 99–116.

or be sent to a hospital for the criminally insane rather than a jail or prison. Or simulation may be used to set the stage for an anticipated plea of insanity. Here the defendant might hope that the court will be convinced that he is insane now and was also insane when the crime was committed. (The defendant can also make no pretense of being mentally ill when examined, but may falsify information in an effort to convince the examiner that he was insane at the time of the crime. This kind of dishonesty relates to the past and does not require the strenuous efforts needed to feign mental illness in the present.)

The astute clinician will often pick up cues that lead him to believe the patient may be malingering. Malingerers, for example, are inclined to overact their parts. The strangeness of their behavior may be far greater than that seen in the usual psychotic patient. Malingerers also try to avoid examination when possible and their condition may change drastically for the better once they realize that simulation is no longer necessary. Psychological tests may also be of value in detecting simulation.

The clinician should be aware that the offender may engage in self-serving irrational behavior without being aware that he is doing so. Such "unconscious malingering" is usually viewed as a form of hysteria and as a bona fide illness. Even more important, the clinician must appreciate that psychotic individuals may also exaggerate symptoms in order to avoid difficult situations. Thus, an offender may be psychotic and malingering at the same time. Some psychiatrists have also noted that a certain number of individuals try to present themselves to others as malingering in order to cover up the existence of a real illness, both to others and to themselves.[17]

All too often the patient whom we think is simulating an illness often turns out to have a severe illness. John McDonald, a prominent forensic psychiatrist, tells the story of a consulting physician who, while walking to his ward one day with his intern, remarked, "Well, how are they all this morning?" "All doing excellently," said the intern, "except the malingerer in the corner who died last night.[18]

The psychiatric examiner is wise simply to note the behaviors he might consider to be evidence of malingering in his report and to be extremely cautious in labeling a patient a malingerer. As a general rule, the court will have a much higher index of suspicion as to the possibility of malingering than the psychiatrist. Even minimal concern on the psychiatrist's part will alert the court as to the possibility of simulation.

[17]S. L. Halleck, *Psychiatry and the Dilemmas of Crime* (New York: Harper, 1967).
[18]J. MacDonald, *Psychiatry and the Criminal* (Springfield, Ill.: Charles C Thomas, 1969), p. 211.

What Is the Relevance of a Defendant's Amnesia in the Incompetency Examination?

Not uncommonly, an offender claims to have no recollection of the period of time in which the crime for which he is charged occurred. There are many possible causes of such amnesia. It may be functional or organic. If functional, it may be genuine or feigned. Functional amnesia is certainly treatable and it would be advantageous to the defendant to be found incompetent until his memory could be restored. In situations where the patient has sustained severe brain damage, however, the possibility of restoration of memory for the alleged criminal event is remote. Organically determined amnesia is not rare among offenders. In crimes associated with violence the offender may himself be harmed, and if his brain is damaged he may have no recollection of the events involved in the crime.

It would seem that the courts would have considerable interest in delaying the trial of amnesic patients, particularly when psychiatric testimony indicates that the amnesia may be reversible. In practice, however, amnesia is given little weight in support of an incompetency plea. The courts fear that there is too much potential for fraudulent allegations of memory loss. In rejecting amnesia as a major criterion of incompetence the courts have argued that the defendants have the opportunity to reconstruct the facts of the case from sources other than their own memory, and that everybody suffers from at least some "amnesia" at various times. It would make some sense for the courts to give patients who claim amnesia some benefit of doubt and to allow for brief postponement of trial. Those amnesics whose memory returned would be benefited by the delay. Neither society nor the patient would be appreciably harmed if patients whose amnesia did not clear up (because of malingering or organicity) were tried just a little later.

How Is the Use of Psychotropic Medication Involved in Determining the Offender's Competency to Stand Trial?

Severely psychotic individuals who might be grossly incapacitated as defendants are frequently restored to a much higher level of mental functioning by psychotropic medication. The proper drug used in the proper dosage may transform the patient from a state of incompetency to one of competency. There is nothing unusual about this. In fact, we ordinarily hope that things work out this way in medicine. When nonpsychotropic drugs are used the courts do not mind dealing with patients whose capacity to participate in the trial is maintained by drugs.

No court would be concerned if a patient who was so physically in-capacitated by heart failure that he was unable to participate in the trial process were made healthy enough to participate by the use of digitalis. For reasons which are not entirely clear, however, the courts have been inconsistent in accepting the competency of patients which is main-tained by psychotropic medication. Some courts have referred to these patients as "synthetically sane" and have insisted that the accused must come to trial in a "natural state."[19] One probable agenda here is that the court is primarily concerned with keeping under control a defendant they assume is dangerous. The courts may fear that the patient made competent by medication might go to trial, be found innocent, be re-leased to the community, stop using his medication, and become "dangerous." Psychiatrists should not support this kind of reasoning. If ever there is a situation in which there is cause for viewing mental disease under a medical model, it is when medication restores mental abilities. Although psychotropic drugs do not restore an individual's health nearly as efficiently as other drugs such as digitalis or insulin, there is not much difference between arguing that the mentally ill per-son should come to court without psychotropic medication and that a diabetic should come to trial without insulin.

There are other situations in which it is the defendant rather than the court or the prosecutor who insists that the medication be stopped during the course of the trial. Some offenders feel, probably incorrectly, that if medicated they will not be able to think clearly during the course of the trial. Other defendants worry that they will look too bizarre. Their attorneys may fear that they may look too calm, particularly in cases where the facts of the crime would normally elicit a strong emotional response. Although defendants are more likely to be harmed than helped by going to trial without the use of medication, there would seem to be no problem in denying them this privilege if they and their attor-neys insist on it.

Are There Ways in Which the Psychiatrist Can Contribute to the Abuse of the Incompetency Process?

By finding too many people incompetent the psychiatrist can con-tribute to increasing the expense of the legal process, can delay justice for some defendants, and may make it easier for others to avoid retribu-tion. When competency examinations are requested by the court or the prosecuting attorney, psychiatrists may also find themselves pawns in a

[19]State v. Murphy, 56 Wash. 2d 761, 355 P.2d 323, 327 (1960).

process in which unconvicted defendants are institutionalized for long periods of time. By failing to insist on briefer periods of confinement for conducting the examination or the use of outpatient examinations of defendants, psychiatrists contribute to the expense of the process and the deprivation of patients' rights. In the potential abuses listed above, psychiatrists are passive participants. Still, if we examine patients and testify about them in court, we are supporting the status quo unless our cooperation is accompanied by vigorous protests against abuses of the incompetency process in public forums.

There is one way in which the psychiatrist might in the course of the examination cause the patient direct harm. During the interview the psychiatrist may discover information that is incriminating to the defendant and include this material in his report. This happens rarely, but it certainly has occurred in states where such information is not privileged. In this situation the psychiatrist falls into a police investigation or prosecutory role. Many states are now initiating legislation which makes any information revealed to the psychiatrist in the course of the competency examination that is relevant to the issue of the crime privileged and inadmissable as evidence in any criminal or civil proceeding.

Abraham Halpern, one of the staunchest critics of the use of the incompetency plea, feels that psychiatrists are misused by the process.[20] He favors abolition of the incompetency plea, but argues that if the psychiatrist does participate in the process he should:

1. Try to participate in the initial screening process when the issue of competency is first raised.
2. Not undertake a competency examination unless the court makes available to the psychiatrist "reasonable grounds" for its opinion that the defendant is incapacitated.
3. Contact the defendant's attorney to learn whether the impending competency examination meets with the attorney's approval. If the defendant's attorney opposes the examination, the psychiatrist may be violating medical ethics by performing it.
4. Try to discover if there is in fact a defense attorney involved. There have been instances in which the court has referred defendants for competency examinations before attorneys were appointed.
5. Try to examine patients sent to hospitals on the day of arrival, and if the decision of competency can be reached at that point, try to return the defendant immediately to the referring court.
6. Insist on being provided a copy of the accusatory instrument

---

[20]Halpern, "Use and Misuse of Psychiatry."

relating to the defendant as well as a copy of the arresting police officer's report. This information is usually necessary to determine whether the defendant understands the charges against him.

7. Work toward returning to court as quickly as possible any defendant found incompetent.
8. Inform the defense attorney immediately if it appears that the patient is unlikely to regain competency so that the attorney can find the most appropriate disposition for the client.[21]

Halpern's suggestions seem quite reasonable and would probably be supported by the majority of psychiatrists who have had extensive experience in dealing with the incompetency plea.

How Long Can a Patient Found Incompetent to Stand Trial Be Kept in an Institution for the Criminally Insane?

Up until 1972 there were no limits in most states on the length of time an incompetent defendant could be kept in a hospital for the criminally insane. There have been many "atrocity cases" in which defendants who were never found guilty of a crime spent the remainder of their lives in a closed institution. In 1972 the Supreme Court ruled in *Jackson v. Indiana* that the incompetency commitment must be temporary and must have some likelihood of being effective in restoring the defendant to competency. The court held that "A person charged . . . with a criminal offense who is committed solely on account of his incapacity to proceed to trial can not be held more than the reasonable period of time necessary to determine whether there is a substantial probability that he will attain that capacity in the foreseeable future. If it is determined that the defendant probably soon will be able to stand trial, his continued commitment must be justified by progress towards that goal."[22] The *Jackson* decision mandates release from commitment to a hospital for the criminally insane when there is no substantial probability that the defendant's condition is treatable. If the defendant is not making progress toward regaining competency, the charges must either be dismissed or he must be civilly committed just like any other individual who is felt to be mentally ill and dangerous.

The *Jackson* court did not specify what a "reasonable period" of commitment might be. Following that decision, however, a number of states have limited the term of commitment to twelve, fifteen, or eigh-

[21]*Ibid.*
[22]Jackson v. Indiana, 406 U.S. 715 (1972).

teen months, or a period not to exceed the maximum sentence for the offense charged.[23] One observer has noted, however, that the *Jackson* limitation on length of confinement is not followed faithfully in all places.[24] Although "atrocities" are unlikely these days, there are still defendants who are in jeopardy of spending several years in a hospital for the criminally insane without having been tried for a crime.

How Treatable Are Defendants Found Incompetent to Stand Trial?

If the goal of treatment is restoring the patient's competency rather than "cure" of the patient's psychosis, the great majority of individuals found incompetent to stand trial could be treated and sent back to court quickly. The majority of defendants carrying diagnoses of schizophrenia, bipolar affective disorder, or psychotic depression, should, if treated in an institution with adequate psychiatric facilities, be sufficiently improved in two to three months (or a much shorter period) to return to court. Only in rare instances should a period of six months or longer be necessary to restore competency.

It is likely that people who have not regained competency within six months will remain permanently incompetent or incompetent for years. Patients with severe mental retardation or organic psychoses are unlikely to regain competency. The eventual disposition of this group can be a cause of concern for society. At first glance it would seem that under the *Jackson* ruling there would be no problem in dealing with patients who never regain competency since those who are nondangerous would simply be released and those who are dangerous would be committed to an ordinary mental hospital. The problem here is that with all the new restrictions governing civil commitment, it is possible that offenders who have probably committed quite serious crimes could not meet the requirements for commitment to a civil hospital. It is often extremely difficult to prove that a patient who has simply been accused of a dangerous act which may have taken place months or years ago is "imminently dangerous" to others. Or a patient may be incompetent for reasons other than mental illness (e.g., a deaf mute) and not meet the mental illness standard of committability.

The model statute of the American Bar Association Commission on the Mentally Disabled requires that there be an alternative of a special commitment proceeding tailored to the situation in which a criminal

---

[23]Ennis, *Prisoners of Psychiatry.*
[24]Halpern, "Use and Misuse of Psychiatry in Competency Examination of Criminal Defendants."

defendant is found unrestorably incompetent to stand trial, but nevertheless represents a substantial threat to inflict serious bodily harm on others.[25] This proposed statute calls for new legal hearings to determine if the patient is indeed dangerous to others insofar as there is substantial evidence that he has committed a serious crime. The criteria for this special commitment would require proof beyond a reasonable doubt that the defendant committed a dangerous offense. Persons who would have been acquitted had they been tried would not be subject to this form of commitment. Although the special type of commitment recommended by the American Bar Association has not been enacted by any legislature, it may become a desirable alternative for states facing the issue of having to release defendants in situations where there is substantial evidence that they have committed dangerous crimes.

What Further Reforms in the Use of the Incompetency Plea Have Been Suggested?

The reforms suggested by psychiatrists have already been noted. These emphasize rapid screening of defendants suspected of incompetency, rapid examination on an outpatient basis where possible, and rapid return to court. Some attorneys have also argued that in certain instances criminal proceedings should be allowed to go forward despite the defendant's incompetency.[26] The Supreme Court made the observation that this might be a reasonable alternative in *Jackson v. Indiana*. The court noted with apparent approval that "some states have statutory provisions permitting pretrial motions to be made or even allowing the incompetent defendant a trial at which to establish his innocence without permitting a conviction."[27] Other attorneys have argued that since the courts have been willing to try patients suffering from permanent amnesia and have also been willing to try in absentia patients who are obviously disruptive, that there may be ways of modifying various court procedures so that even permanently incompetent defendants can receive a fair trial.[28] At its extreme, this argument takes the form of a demand for the abolition of the incompetency plea. Although it would seem that the Supreme Court in earlier decisions has insisted on the

[25]Commission on the Mentally Disabled, American Bar Association, "Suggested Statute on Incompetence to Stand Trial on Criminal Charges," *Mental Disability Law Reporter 2*, no. 5 (1978): 636–50.

[26]Ennis, *Prisoners of Psychiatry.*

[27]Jackson v. Indiana, 406 U.S. 715, (1972).

[28]B. Ennis and C. Hansen, "Memorandum of Law: Competence to Stand Trial, "*Journal of Psychiatry and Law*, Winter 1976, pp. 491–514.

retention of the incompetency plea, some legal scholars have insisted that with sufficient changes in procedural rules, the incapacities and disadvantages suffered by an incompetent defendant could be largely remedied and that all incompetent defendants could be tried.[29]

Even though there is much criticism of the incompetency plea, the psychiatrist should not anticipate great reform in this area in the near future. What we are likely to see is some broadening of the category of defendants who are found competent to stand trial, more rapid assessments of competency in less restrictive settings, and perhaps new laws which create a means of providing custody of dangerous but permanently incompetent offenders.

[29]R. Burt and N. Morris, "A Proposal for the Abolition of the Incompetency Plea, "*University of Chicago Law Review 40,* no. 60 (1972): 77–79.

13

Child Custody

Divorce has an obvious and dramatic effect on the children of the dissolved union. In addition to all the other traumas involved in the dissolution process, the child must face a situation in which the availability and nurturance of both parents will be severely curtailed. As a rule divorce results in the child's living with one or the other parent. That parent is given custody of the child, which means that he or she is responsible for the welfare, health, and control of that child. The other parent may see the child infrequently or not at all. In the majority of divorces, the parents are able to resolve the issue of their children's custody more or less amicably. Not infrequently, however, both parents demand custody of the child. When parents cannot resolve this dispute on their own, the issue must be settled in court.

The emotional issues involved in custody battles for children are powerful, and battles for custody are likely to be vicious. Most marriages are terminated in an atmosphere of anger and bitterness. Separation may be accompanied by relentless battles over property as well as children. In such a situation the child is in jeopardy of being used to satisfy certain parental needs. Parents, for example, may demand custody of the child as a threat or maneuver to force the spouse to provide a more generous property settlement. The child may be demanded by a parent who is not really interested in raising that child, but is primarily interested in making life as difficult and unrewarding as possible for the ex-spouse. Even in states such as California which have instituted a no-fault divorce system which allows couples to separate amicably, child custody disputes are fought as viciously as ever. In fact, it is possible that hard-fought disputes are more likely under a no-fault system since spouses who previously might have given up custody demands in order to find an easy way out of a marriage no longer have to do so.

One forensic psychiatrist has referred to child custody cases as the "ugliest litigation."[1] These cases tend to be shunned by successful attorneys and to be viewed with apprehension by juvenile and family court judges. When the court is faced with the momentous decision as to which parent should obtain custody of the child, it is entirely understandable that the judge would be concerned with the mental well-being of the child and the mental health of both parents in the dispute, and would seek expert advice about these issues. Psychiatrists, particularly child psychiatrists, are welcomed to participate in child custody disputes as experts, and distasteful as this work may be for all concerned, a substantial number of psychiatrists are willing to assist the courts in this area.

What Changes in Legal Doctrine Have Been Especially Significant in Resolving Child Custody Disputes?

The law and practices with regard to child custody have changed drastically in the last two centuries, and some of the problems related to determination of custody become a little clearer when viewed in a historical perspective. From the time of the Roman empire and through the middle ages, fathers were given absolute control over their children. When marriages collapsed, the children automatically went to the father on the assumption that they were his personal property. Whenever parents lived apart and there was a dispute over custody, the right of the father automatically took precedence over that of the mother.[2]

By the beginning of the nineteenth century, the English courts began to reflect the prevailing social ethos that custody involved not only rights but also responsibilities for the care of the child. Under the *parens patriae* doctrine, child custody became an important issue in courts of law and in some situations custody was awarded to the mother.[3] Throughout most of the nineteenth century, however, most cases brought to litigation in the United States resulted in the award of custody to the father.

Even in the nineteenth century, a number of decisions began to reflect a change toward favoring granting custody to the mother. This change was first initiated with regard to young children. It was assumed that a child of "very tender years" needed the care and attention of a mother, at least until the child reached the age where the father could

---

[1]M. G. Goldzband, "Child Custody: The Ugliest Litigation: A Guarded Word of Welcome," *Bulletin of the American Academy of Psychiatry and Law* 4, no. 3 (1976): 101–104.
[2]J. Areen, *Family Law* (Mineola, N.Y.: Foundation Press, 1978).
[3]A. P. Derdeyn, "Child Custody Contests in Historical Perspective," *American Journal of Psychiatry* 133, no. 12 (1976): 1369–76.

offer it proper care. By the end of the nineteenth century, when women were gaining new rights and children were being accorded more attention, the tendency to provide custody to the mother was strengthened.[4] There was a distinct shift from the father's having total control, to both parties' being equal contestants, to the mother's having the paramount claim to the child.

In the latter part of the nineteenth and the early part of the twentieth century, court decisions began to emphasize the *parens patriae* responsibility of the courts to do what is best for the interests of the child. Gradually these decisions have evolved into a doctrine now reinforced by statute in most states which emphasizes that the custody placement must be in the best interests of the child. It appears that the best interests of the child standard initially developed in order to further the doctrine of allowing the child to be placed with the mother. Indeed, throughout this century there has been an ever-increasing tendency to award custody rights to mothers, and in the 1960s, 90% of these cases were decided in favor of the mother.

The best interests of the child doctrine is an elusive one. What is best for the child usually reflects prevailing opinions regarding the status of men and women with regard to childrearing. The state may have a *parens patriae* commitment to look out for the child's interests, but it cannot avoid paying careful attention to the pleas of both parents, both of whom feel that placement of the child with them is in the best interest of the child. Up until the 1970s, the courts tended to rely rather heavily on social customs and moral standards in determining best interests placements. In the 1970s, we have seen much more equality between the sexes, and many customary assumptions as to what is best for a child are being questioned. In a society characterized by rapid change, the best interests doctrine is subject to a variety of interpretations. As legal and social criteria for making custody decisions are losing specificity, the judge is provided with greater discretion. In large part, this discretion is unwelcomed. Many judges are now eager and willing to seek the expert assistance of psychiatrists in deciding on the agonizing issue of custody.

What Is the Legal Setting in Which Child Custody Cases Are Heard?

In the majority of instances child custody disputes are between a husband and wife in the process of divorce. The issue of custody may also arise in other proceedings involving adoption and guardianship.

[4]R. Shepherd, "Solomon's Sword: Adjudication of Child Custody Questions," *University of Richmond Law Review* 8 (1974): 151–200.

Disputes may also be between different groups of relatives or between nonrelatives and natural parents. All these cases are resolved by the decision of a judge instead of a jury.

Child custody cases are decided by the traditional adversary system. Commonly, each parent in the dispute will hire an attorney to help argue his or her case. The adversarial system would seem to be most appropriate here as long as one considers children to be possessions or a form of property. But once the legal doctrine changes to the best interests of the child, the issue of whether such a doctrine can be served by a battle between two parents becomes muddled. It is the child's interests that are at stake, but the battle is actually fought between two other parties, each of whom claims to represent the child's interests. Some courts have tried to resolve this problem by appointing an attorney to represent the interests of the child. This practice has had only limited effectiveness since the attorney representing the child's interests is, in effect, faced with the same problems as the judge. He, too, must listen to the adversaries in the proceeding and decide which makes the better case for the child's custody.

Appeals in child custody cases are available, as in most legal processes, but they are relatively uncommon. There must be a clear abuse of the judge's discretion before an appeal is generally allowed. While initial decisions are rarely appealed, changes in custody can be granted at a later date if there is a "substantial change in circumstances." Thus, parents who lose the initial decision can often find a basis for relitigating the issue, particularly in a different jurisdiction. Some psychiatrists have argued that the constant pursuit of the "best environment" for the child can have destructive consequences in the custody decision to the extent that it keeps the custody decision from becoming final.[5] They note that it is extremely difficult for the parent awarded custody to develop a spontaneous relationship with the child when there is a constant danger that the custody arrangement may be challenged and disrupted. They believe that once the custodial decision is made, it should be extremely difficult, if not impossible, to reopen the issue. Other psychiatrists take a more flexible position.

In Actual Practice, What Kinds of Issues Are Considered in Meeting the "Best Interests" Standards?

Although judicial discretion in this area is increasing, it is probably still true that the majority of decisions are heavily influenced by prece-

---

[5] A. Watson, "The Children of Armageden: Problems of Custody Following Divorce," *Syracuse Law Review* 2, no. 55 (1969): 80.

dent and by social prejudices. In the overwhelming number of cases, for example, young children, particularly young girls, will be awarded to the custody of the mother. There is a tendency to allow fathers to have custody of older boys. When there is more than one child, efforts are usually made to keep them in the same home. The value systems of parents continue to play a role in custody decisions. Parents who adhere to lifestyles (for example, homosexuality) which do not meet with the approval of the majority of the community are at a distinct disadvantage in obtaining custody of children.[6] Even though mothers are generally favored in the majority of custody decisions, a lesbian mother is not likely to be a successful contestant.

Value systems are usually only one variable considered in determining the fitness of a parent to have custody. The capacity of the parent to provide the child with the material needs which will favor his welfare may also be an important consideration in resolving a dispute. The health of the parents is another issue. While mental illness does not automatically disqualify a parent from obtaining custody, it is a factor that is considered. The parent who has been mentally ill must often go to considerable lengths to obtain testimony attesting to his or her current health. Any kind of past criminality will obviously weaken a given parent's case for custody. At one time adultery, particularly on the part of a wife, substantially strengthened the husband's argument for custody. Today this issue is still considered, but it exerts far less powerful influence than it once did. Where the sexual indiscretions of the parent are known to the child, the fact of adultery is likely to exercise more weight in the custody decision than otherwise. As has been noted earlier, all the above-listed precedents and moral guidelines are beginning to be questioned, and although they still exert considerable influence in most jurisdictions, they are providing much less clear direction for the judge.

How Important Is the Child's Preference in the Court's Decision?

Often the child will have some preference as to which parent he wishes to live with. As might be expected, the extent to which the child's preference influences the custody decision varies directly with the child's age. An adolescent's preference will logically have more influence than that of a five- or six-year-old child. Even the firmly expressed preference of an older child, however, will not fully determine the court's decision. The court must consider the possibility that the child does not know what is best for him and may be indicating the wrong

[6]B. Harris, "Lesbian Mother Child Custody: Legal and Psychiatric Aspects," *Bulletin of the American Academy of Psychiatry and the Law 5,* no. 1 (1977): 75–90.

preference. It is also possible that the child is under considerable pressure from one parent or another to indicate a preference. Some child psychiatrists have argued that it may be extremely traumatic to ask younger children to indicate a preference.[7] The child may feel that he is hurting or rejecting the parent he does not select and that he may later be rejected by that parent. Many judges will talk to children in their chambers and try to elicit the child's preference. Some attorneys will use knowledge of the child's preference in arguing their cases. It has also been argued that in situations where the child has a lawyer appointed to represent his interests, the lawyer may have a responsibility to advocate the child's indicated preference. Such a doctrine must be based on a belief that the child is competent to choose in his own best interests.

How Does the Psychiatrist Usually Get Involved in Child Custody Proceedings?

Sometimes the psychiatrist is asked by the court to help determine the best interests of the child. In other instances, the attorneys for both parents may agree to enlist the same psychiatrist's services and compromise their adversarial position. In a typical case, however, the psychiatrist is called by one side or the other to do the evaluation.

Most psychiatrists who become involved in child custody disputes prefer to avoid the adversarial position, arguing that if they are truly to serve the best interests of the child they should not be the advocate of either parent.[8] Some psychiatrists who testify regularly in these kinds of cases have devised interesting techniques for avoiding the adversarial stance. When called by the lawyer for one or another parent, the psychiatrist may insist that he will not take the case unless both lawyers agree to employ him and to make some commitment to be influenced by his decision. Other psychiatrists may even insist that parents agree to be bound by the psychiatrist's recommendation. (The argument here is that psychiatrists know more about determining the best interests of the child than the court, and that while any decision has to be approved through a legal process, psychiatric input into this process must be given critical influence.)

The attempt of psychiatrists to break out of the adversarial mold

---

[7]A. M. Levy, "Child Custody Determination—a Proposed Psychiatric Methdology and Its Resultant Case Typology," *Journal of Psychiatry and Law,* Summer 1978, pp. 189–214.

[8]R. Solow and P. Adams, "Custody by Agreement: Child Psychiatrist as Child Advocate," *Journal of Psychiatry and Law,* Spring 1977, pp. 77–101; T. A. Rodgers, "The Crisis of Custody: How a Psychiatrist Can Be of Help," *Bulletin of the American Academy of Psychiatry and the Law 4,* no. 3 (1976): 114–19.

with regard to the child custody issue is in many ways justifiable and rational. This type of litigation does not ideally lend itself to an adversarial approach. The best interests of the child are unlikely to be served when his parents engage in a furious battle over his custody. Even when psychiatrists function as agents of one parent or another, they do tend to try to obtain as broad a picture of the situation as possible. This means that they try to examine both parents as well as the child. Both parents in litigation must usually consent to such an examination since a failure to do so might be viewed by the judge as seriously compromising their case.

What Steps Does the Psychiatrist Usually Take in Formulating an Opinion in Child Custody Cases?

The psychiatrist who testifies in child custody disputes should be exceptionally deliberate and thorough. More experienced psychiatrists who work in this area usually try to obtain a court directive or an agreement between both attorneys which allows them to examine all concerned parties. As a rule, both parents are interviewed separately. All involved children are examined. Some psychiatrists insist on conjoint interviews between children with parents and conjoint interviews with the parents alone. All this is time-consuming and expensive, and usually requires very precise prearrangement for compensating for the psychiatrist's time.

In the course of their examination, psychiatrists are attempting to evaluate the strengths and weaknesses of all concerned parties. They are particularly concerned with the parenting abilities of the parties in litigation, with their capacity to provide psychological nurturance, with their capacity to communicate, and with the degree to which they are in "tune" with the child. Evaluation of the child and the child's needs, of course, usually requires some skill in child psychiatry. As a general rule, the doctor who involves himself in child custody proceedings should be a child psychiatrist or should have considerable training in this field.

If the psychiatrist becomes involved in an adversarial role where it is only possible for him to examine the child and one of the parents involved in the controversy, the psychiatrist's opinion will obviously have less weight. Here his conclusory statements about the best interests of the child should be made much more cautiously. When the psychiatrist does not examine one of the parents in the controversy, he really has no way of evaluating that parent's fitness to raise the child. He should be extremely careful to avoid making statements that are critical of that individual's capacity. Generally, when only one parent has been examined the psychiatrist is wise to focus on the strengths of that parent and the advantages the child might experience in living with that parent.

How Valuable Are the Psychiatrists' Contributions in Child Custody Disputes?

The testimony of psychiatrists in a child custody dispute probably has much more influence on the court's decision than in most other situations where the psychiatrist testifies as an expert. In this area it makes good sense for the psychiatrist to present conclusory opinions and for the courts to listen to them because the standard of "best interests of the child" is as much a psychological one as a legal one. The psychiatrist is dealing with an extremely difficult question but at least it is one about which he, in theory, has some expertise. His statements should be conclusory, and in those situations where he functions as a neutral witness rather than as a pure adversary, his recommendations are likely to be accepted.

Yet we would be grandiose if we did not admit to having powerful limitations of our capacity to determine the child's best interests. Psychiatrists are really not very skilled at predicting the future behavior of anyone, and while we can sometimes argue with considerable certainty that a particular living situation will be harmful to a child, in more equivocal situations we cannot predict the long-term result to the child. We should also be aware that in addition to being professionals, we are also ordinary citizens who are deeply influenced by the morality of our community. We have value systems that will often influence our determination of what is "healthy" and what is "unhealthy." In the absence of any absolute data as to what is the "best" method of childrearing, we all have our prejudices which will influence our determination as to who might be the best parent. The testimony of many psychiatrists in child custody disputes suggests that they are not immune from being heavily influenced by prevailing moralistic attitudes in the community. There is no scientific evidence that adherence to such attitudes leads to outcomes in the best interests of the child.

In What Situations Other Than Divorce of Natural Parents May the Psychiatrist Be Called upon to Assist in Determining Custody Disputes of Children?

Sometimes disputes over child custody do not involve parents who are in the process of divorce but will involve other parties. There have been a number of controversial cases in which the grandparents of the child have sought custody after one of the parents has died.[9] Or a step-parent who may have been raising the child may ask for custody when the natural parent dies or seeks a divorce. These cases are every bit as complicated, if not more so, than the disputes between natural parents, and frequently call for the same type of thorough evaluation by a psychiatrist.

Sometimes the rights of parents to custody of a child are terminated and children are given to the custody of the state. Parental rights can be terminated when there are conditions present which have produced serious substantial and continuous damage to the health and welfare of a child. The court must also determine that termination of parental rights is in the best interests of the child. Again, thorough psychiatric evaluation may be of considerable value to the courts in making such decisions.

Each year in the United States, between one hundred and two hundred thousand children are brought before the courts on the grounds that they are being neglected or abused by their parents. Once the court assumes jurisdiction in order to protect the child, it can separate the child from his family for months, for years, or permanently. There is much disagreement from jurisdiction to jurisdiction as to when a child should be defined as neglected or abused, and even when such a determination has been made there is little consensus as to when the child should be removed from the parental home. There are obviously considerable disadvantages to the emotional welfare of the child when he is removed from his parents. On the other hand, if the home appears to be one in which the child will inevitably suffer physical and emotional damage, the obligation of the state to protect the child seems clear.

Although testimony before the courts on child abuse and neglect cases is most likely to be provided by social workers, psychiatrists may also be requested to assess the mental stability of the child and the parents, and to try to make predictions as to whether the child's emotional well-being will be endangered by remaining in the parental home. Many psychiatrists these days feel that except in instances where there is extreme abuse (such as regular beatings of children or sexual molestation) or extreme neglect (which endangers the child's physical health), efforts should be made to try to work with the family to improve their parenting skills.[10] The emphasis on "rehabilitating" the family rather than removing the child from the home is based on the belief that par-

[9]Painter v. Bannister, 258 Iowa 1390, 140 N.W.2d 152 (1966).

[10]S. L. Halleck, "Violence in Families," *Continuing Education for the Family Physician 9*, no. 5 (1978): 26–39.

ents can be taught childrearing skills, can receive counseling for their own problems, and can learn to do better. Psychiatrists have also been active in urging that temporary placements be developed to care for children for brief periods of time while parents are dealing with personal crises in their own lives.

14

The Psychiatrist's Role in Evaluating Psychic Injury

The role of stress as a determinant of psychiatric symptomatology is well documented.[1] Variables related to an individual's preexisting biological and psychological vulnerabilities will, of course, play a key role in determining if he is damaged by a particular stress. But a recent stress itself is usually a partial and necessary cause of most emotional disorders. The law is not designed to provide remedies for individuals who may be damaged by the ordinary stresses of everyday life. It has, however, paid considerable attention to damage created by the behavior of individuals who are at fault and stress another person, either intentionally or through negligent conduct.

The law recognizes that damages may have a psychic component. Mental suffering is usually considered as one element in determining compensation for individuals damaged in an automobile accident as the result of someone's negligence. It is also an element in determining compensation for damages resulting from the negligent malpractice of doctors. In those few recorded cases where negligent psychotherapy has been proven, for example, the main basis for awards has been the psychic injury imposed on the patient. For a variety of historical reasons, the law has also become concerned with psychic damages created by stressful conditions related to work. Work-related accidents or diseases are compensable in all states through Workmen's Compensation laws.

Suits based on psychic injury are increasing. This may be a spin-off effect from the new legalism and "lawsuit consciousness" of society, but changing perspectives as to the nature of psychiatric illness may also

---

[1]L. Yochelson, "Traumatic Neurosis," in *Readings in Law and Psychiatry*, edited by R. C. Allen *et al.* (Baltimore: Johns Hopkins University Press, 1975), pp. 452–60; H. C. Modlin, "The Trauma in 'Traumatic Neurosis,'" *Bulletin of the Menninger Clinic* 24 (1960): 49–56; K. Menninger, *The Vital Balance* (New York: Viking Press, 1963).

account for some of the change. In recent years, society and the courts have come to be somewhat more accepting of psychiatry. People believe that psychic injuries occur and that patients who claim that they are experiencing emotional suffering are not simply malingering. More than that, there seems to be an increasing belief that advances in psychiatry have made it possible for psychiatrists to provide the court with information as to which patients who experience psychic distress are malingering and which should be thought of as sick.

What Is the Role of the Psychiatrist in Personal Injury Evaluation?

As a general rule, a psychiatrist testifies as to the degree of psychiatric damage that has taken place as a result of stresses emanating from work conditions or from the tortious behavior of others. In addition to testifying as to the nature and extent of damage, the psychiatrist is also expected to make some statements regarding causation, that is, how work-related conditions or stresses created by faults of others have produced damages. Traditionally, the courts have been so suspicious of the concept of psychic injuries that plaintiffs have not received awards unless the psychic damages were the result of some kind of physical injury, or at least physical impact or touching.[2] The courts, for example, have little difficulty in understanding how one who incurred serious facial scarring as a result of an accident might easily experience psychic trauma. But they have been much more reluctant to find that psychic stresses can produce psychic injuries. Until recently, suits alleging that psychic injury followed from psychic stress (such as witnessing a horrible accident) were not compensable. This situation is changing rapidly.[3] Particularly under Workmen's Compensation laws, we are now seeing an increasing number of awards for psychic injury based on psychic trauma.

It is also conceivable, of course, that psychic trauma including work-related or tortious-related stress can also produce physical injury through psychophysiologic processes. We are seeing more cases in which awards are granted in situations in which plaintiffs develop ulcers and other physiologic ailments under highly stressful conditions.[4] In

[2]R. Slovenko, *Psychiatry and Law* (Boston: Little, Brown, 1973), p. 295.
[3]J. Robitscher, "The Uses and Abuses of Psychiatry, Lecture I," *Journal of Psychiatry and Law*, Fall 1977, pp. 333–66.
[4]N. Brill and J. Glass, "Workmen's Compensation for Psychiatric Disorders," *Journal of the American Medical Association 193*, no. 5 (1965): 345–48.

evaluating these cases, the psychiatrist does not usually testify as to the extent of the damages which are more "physical" than "psychic," but may be asked to give an opinion as to how certain stresses were factors in causing the psychophysiologic disorder.

In Workmen's Compensation actions, the psychiatrist may be employed by a state agency to estimate the patient's disability and present his findings before a relatively informal board. In most instances, the findings are accepted and the case does not go to a more formal tribunal. If the case is not settled, however, the worker who is the plaintiff and the employer or his insurance company each call on their own medical experts to testify as to the extent of the disability. Psychiatrists can end up working for either the plaintiff or the defendant. In suits based on tort actions, the psychiatrist is usually enlisted by either the plaintiff or the defendant while the case is being prepared. A final manner in which psychiatrists might become involved in evaluating psychic injury is in situations involving insurance compensation for psychiatric disability where the insurance company argues that the disorder either does not exist, is not covered by the policy, or was a preexisting condition. These kind of situations, however, are far less frequent than those involving psychic injury related to Workmen's Compensation or tortious behavior.

What Is Workmen's Compensation, and What Is Required of the Psychiatrist Who Testifies in Workmen's Compensation Suits?

Under the common law, it is extremely difficult for an employee to sue his employer. This is because of long-standing legal doctrines denying compensation when injury is caused by a fellow employee (fellow-servant rule), when the patient knew that he was assuming certain risks (assumption of risk rule), or when the worker in some way contributed to his own injury (contributory negligence rule).[5] Around the turn of the century, industrial accidents were common and Workmen's Compensation laws were developed primarily to provide social protection to workers who might be injured but who could not sue their employers. The states developed these statutes with the belief that industrial accidents could be insured so that workmen could be protected from interruption of income and could be provided with adequate medical care and rehabilitation. These statutes require employers to carry insurance which compensates job-related injuries whether the employer was at fault or not. Workmen's Compensation laws are also designed to encourage

[5]T. E. Carrol, "Workmen's Compensation: A Senile Form of Social Insurance," *Journal of Rehabilitation* 35 (1968): 15.

employers to work toward creating the safest possible work environments.

Workmen's Compensation disputes differ from tort litigation primarily in that as they are not based on fault. It does not matter if the employer was or was not negligent when the employee was injured: the employee can still receive some award. As a general rule, however, awards based on Workmen's Compensation are not nearly as high as they are in tort law. The laws are designed primarily to protect the worker's income over a limited period of time, and at best he usually receives a percentage of his salary over that period of time.

The physician's task in a Workmen's Compensation case is to find damages and to show how they might be caused by work-related conditions. Here the physician must also estimate the extent of disability. This is often a difficult task, and formulas which assist the physician at arriving at an estimate may vary from state to state.

Over the years there has been a tendency for Workmen's Compensation boards and the courts to provide awards not only for accidents related to direct trauma but also for diseases related to more subtle and insidious work stress. Most state laws now cover both work-related diseases and accidents. There is concern among some authorities that Workmen's Compensation is being used in too liberal a manner as a form of sickness insurance.[6] This concern is fueled by the realization that there are far fewer accidents and injuries than there used to be and yet Workmen's Compensation claims are increasing. Many of these claims are based on psychic injury. The possibility that psychic stress will become a plausible explanation of psychic disability which will justify granting the plaintiff awards leads some commentators to wonder whether such cases will proliferate endlessly and put an unfair burden on the employer.[7]

What Is the Role of the Psychiatrist in Testifying as to Psychic Damages in Cases Based on Tort Law?

As noted in the first section of this book, there may be a mental or motivational element involved in torts which are intentional. An individual who severely distresses another through assault, defamation, or false imprisonment may be liable. Here the psychological consequences of such actions may be so obvious that expert witnesses are not needed.

[6]M. Franklin, *Tort Law and Alternatives* (Mineola, N.Y.: Foundation Press, 1971), chap. 7.
[7]Brill and Glass, "Workmen's Compensation."

As a rule, the psychiatrist becomes involved as an expert only when damages are alleged to have been caused by negligence. Although the great majority of cases in this area involve accidents in which the plaintiff experiences concurrent physical trauma, mental trauma has also been invoked as a sole cause of damages. Awards, for example, have been given in situations where the plaintiff may have witnessed the negligent infliction of physical injury upon a loved one and was thereby traumatized.[8] In obvious cases of grave disability or disfigurement following an accident, some lawyers will prefer to dispense with psychiatric experts in proving psychic damages. They feel that the plaintiff's own testimony and the jury's opportunity to observe the plaintiff provide sufficient evidence of the extent of psychic distress without the need for experts. When expert witnesses are called, however, they are required, as in Workmen's Compensation cases, to describe the extent of damages and the manner in which these damages are related to the injury.

In tort cases and in Workmen's Compensation cases which have gone on to an adversarial process, the psychiatrist will find that his relationship to the patient is somewhat different depending on whether he is employed by the plaintiff or the defendant. When working for the plaintiff, the psychiatrist is likely to find a cooperative patient and should have little difficulty in establishing rapport. When working for the defendant, the psychiatrist may find an unfriendly patient who is distrustful and who might be prone to exaggerate the extent of damages and the severity of stress to which the damages are related. It is relatively easy for the doctor's own value system to color his perception of the patient's disability. Doctors who are more committed to the work ethic and less committed to understanding symptomatology in terms of unconscious motivation may find themselves more comfortable in testifying for the defendant. Psychiatrists more sympathetic to the goals of social welfare and more comfortable with viewing disability based on unconscious motivation as a true illness will be more comfortable in testifying for the plaintiff. A psychiatrist who evaluates personal injuries should be familiar with his personal biases, should acknowledge them to the attorney who employs him, and should strive to keep these biases out of his conclusions and reports. The psychiatrist who always finds himself on one side or the other of this type of litigation should begin to question his commitment to scrupulously scientific testimony, and can anticipate that if he does not question his commitment, opposing attorneys soon will.

[8]"Annotation: Right to Recover Damages in Negligence for Fear of Injury to Another or Shock or Mental Anguish at Witnessing Such Injury," 29 A.L.R.3d 1337 (1970).

What Legal Issues Regarding Causation and Damages Should the Psychiatrist Be Aware of in Examining the Patient?

One of the most perplexing issues for psychiatrists who become involved in psychic injury suits (whether in Workmen's Compensation or tort law) involves trying to relate the extent of damage to a particularly stressful circumstance or set of circumstances. Psychiatric theory is based on multicausality. We rarely view one or even a series of events as a cause of a given disability. Sometimes we can say that a given event may be a "precipitant" of a disorder, but even this kind of term implies some kind of preexisting individual vulnerability or susceptibility. We know that different individuals respond to similar stresses differently and in our usual thinking about patients we avoid ascribing a given behavior to a single cause.

The courts, however, cannot afford such scientific detachment. They must assess blame. There is a tendency for the courts to look upon the precipitating cause of a disorder as the legal cause even if the person had a great deal of preexisting difficulty. Thus, a negligent person is usually liable even if the damages were partly caused by preexisting conditions. It is not until the court assesses damages that it considers the patient's preexisting susceptibility to stress. A person, for example, who is already slightly disabled but who then experiences serious psychic damage as a result of an accident is likely to receive less compensatory damages than a plaintiff who had no preexisting disability.

Psychiatrists have tried to respond to the legal problems involved in evaluating psychic injury be developing classifications of injury-related disorders.[9] In some classifications, the psychiatrist may state that the trauma is a necessary and sufficient cause of the damages, in others a necessary or precipitating cause, and in still others no cause at all. Or the trauma may be viewed as simply aggravating a preexisting condition. These classifications are, in my opinion, unnecessary. Rather than trying to conceptualize the relationship of the trauma to the injury in terms of categories, the psychiatrist would do better meticulously to describe the nature or any preexisting disability and the nature of the plaintiff's personality, and to speculate on how these factors interacted with the stressful circumstances in a manner which may or may not have led to psychic injury. Diagnostic classifications are not nearly as important here as excellent description and dynamic formulation. The psychiatrist may wish to make a conclusive statement that the damage was caused by the trauma, but this is not necessary. It is well to remember that it is the judge or jury who will determine legal causation. The psychiatrist

[9]P. Davidson, *Forensic Psychiatry* (New York: Ronald Press, 1952).

who sticks to his own area of expertise and does not try to stretch causal linkages beyond his data will usually spare himself painful cross-examination.

What Is the Role of Classical Psychiatric Diagnosis in Assessing Damages?

Judges and juries will be more likely to appreciate that psychic damages exist if such damages can be described as emotional disorders which can be classified and labeled. If the patient's disability cannot be classified or labeled, it is more easily dismissed as malingering. The psychiatrist who testifies for the plaintiff is under some pressure to put a name to the patient's disability. Where there has been damage to the brain following an accident, it is relatively easy to characterize the plaintiff's disability with a conventional diagnosis. Sometimes the patient responds to stress with classical symptoms of psychosis or depression and again the labeling problem here is not too complicated. There is also, however, a constellation of symptoms which frequently follow traumatic events and which are more difficult to label. Not infrequently, the patient exposed to severe stress experiences recurring symptoms of irritability, hyperalertness, free-floating anxiety, insomnia, impairment of memory and concentration, withdrawal, agitation, and some reexperiencing of trauma through dreams, fugue states, or somnambulism.[10] This cluster of symptoms has been given a variety of labels, the most common of which is "traumatic neurosis." There is much concern among psychiatrists as to whether this diagnosis has the same authenticity as more classical diagnoses.

Part of our uncertainty with the diagnosis of traumatic neurosis relates to the manner in which its symptoms may be influenced by environmental circumstances which follow the traumatic event, particularly by the reality of impending litigation. Severe stress can produce symptoms of traumatic neurosis in previously normal individuals. Motivations outside the patient's awareness may, however, create and perpetuate symptoms. The patient may, for example, unconsciously perpetuate the symptomatology of a traumatic neurosis in order to obtain an award. Or unconscious motivations to gain sympathy from relatives or revenge against the tortfeasor may have a similar effect. Most psychiatrists believe that where symptoms are perpetuated because of mental processes outside of the patient's awareness, the symptoms are

---

[10]J. B. Robitscher, *Pursuit of Agreement: Psychiatry and the Law* (Philadelphia: Lippincott, 1966).

just as painful and incapacitating as those created by physical impairment. They have little problem in viewing traumatic neurosis as a disease. But other psychiatrists and most laypersons are more skeptical. They are more likely to view symptoms motivated by desires to gain money, sympathy, or revenge as malingering, whether the motivations are conscious or unconscious.

As of this writing, neither the term "traumatic neurosis" nor its many synonyms has been given a place in our standardized diagnostic system. The psychiatrist who uses the term should be prepared to define it on the basis of material he has read in the forensic literature. He must be willing to acknowledge that no such diagnosis appears in *DSM II*, and must be prepared to have his testimony questioned vigorously.

The psychiatrist may encounter similar problems when he uses any diagnosis which implies that the patient's symptoms are determined by unconscious motivations of gain. Some patients do develop symptoms which mimic physical disorders following trauma, but which are not associated with anatomical or physiological dysfunction. These patients are usually described as suffering from dissociative reactions. The diagnosis of dissociative reaction is included in *DSM II*, but the psychiatric expert witness should expect to have its legitimacy questioned. He may have a difficult time arguing that such a patient is not malingering.

In What Way Might DSM III Help in Diagnosing Emotional Disorders Following Trauma?

DSM III, which will soon become the official nomenclature system of the American Psychiatric Association, lists a specific diagnostic category of posttraumatic stress disorder.[11] In order to make this diagnosis the physician must observe a high degree of relatively unusual stress which is severe enough so that it would be likely to produce symptoms in most people. Ordinary stresses such as failure in work or school cannot be included. The symptoms which characterize the posttraumatic stress disorder are similar to those which have described traumatic neurosis. *DSM III* puts considerable emphasis on reexperiencing of trauma, "psychic numbing" or withdrawal, excessive autonomic arousal, and concentration and memory impairment.

One problem with this new diagnostic category is that it requires the physician to make an assessment that the stress the plaintiff experienced is so severe that it would produce symptoms in most people. There

[11]Task Force on Nomenclature and Statistics, American Psychiatric Association, "DSM III—Draft" (Washington, D.C.: APA, 1978).

is considerable literature which indicates that most people do experience symptoms following severe trauma. [12] The requirement of a severe stress, however, might exclude cases in which minor stress elicits major symptomatology. Not infrequently, minor stresses which would not have bothered most people do produce major responses in others.

DSM III also contains a category of malingering. As a rule it is not too difficult to distinguish a posttraumatic stress disorder (as defined in *DSM III*) from malingering. The symptoms of posttraumatic stress disorder are relatively specific and time limited. When the symptoms are chronic, they are of a degree of severity which would be hard for any individual to simulate for a long period of time. There is a much greater problem in distinguishing certain dissociative reactions (called somatiform disorders in *DSM III*) from malingering. *DSM III* advises that the distinction be made on the basis that the patient who has a somatization or conversion (somatiform) disorder does not perceive his symptoms as being under voluntary control, whereas the malingerer does.

Much has been written about the manner in which a psychiatrist can detect malingering, and the courts have some belief that we are gaining greater skill in this area. I am skeptical that this is so. *DSM III* does, however, provide certain guidelines in diagnosing malingering. The malingerer, according to this document, is likely to be an unfriendly patient. He demonstrates a high degree of distress which he always relates to his symptomatology. His symptoms are not likely to be presented in the context of emotional conflict and the psychiatrist usually cannot interpret their symbolic meaning. Finally, his symptoms are not likely to be relieved by suggestion, by hypnosis, or by intravenous barbituate injection.

In summary, *DSM III* is a document which the psychiatrist can cite in diagnosing stress-related disabilities and in distinguishing them from malingering. Using *DSM III* diagnoses may strengthen the credibility the psychiatrist's testimony. The psychiatrist, however, should not become too preoccupied with labeling the patient's disorder. Ultimately, the court will be much more impressed by the accuracy of the psychiatrist's description of the phenomenology and psychodynamics of the disorder than by his use of diagnostic classifications.

[12] A. J. Glass, "Observations upon the Epidemiology of Mental Illness," in "Trends During Warfare," in *Symposium on Preventative and Social Psychiatry* (Washington, D.C.: U.S. Government Printing Office, 1957).

15

Miscellaneous Expert Witness Roles in the Civil Courts

In addition to assisting in child custody disputes and evaluation of psychic damages, the psychiatrist may be asked to assume the following roles in the civil courts:

1. The assessment of an individual's competency to manage business affairs, to make contracts, to make a will, to be a witness, or to marry.
2. The evaluation of the degree of mental illness of an individual who is being sued.
3. The assessment of the mental status of parties in conflict over divorce.
4. Providing expert testimony for either the defendant or plaintiff in a medical malpractice suit.
5. Providing information regarding the psychological effects of repressive practices in suits involving the civil rights of certain classes of individuals such as mental patients who are prisoners.

In most of the above-listed roles, the psychiatrist is permitted, and usually requested, to make conclusory statements. When the psychiatrist testifies in conclusory terms, he must usually make an intellectual leap from medical data to a legal conclusion. Here, as is the case in testimony before the criminal courts, it would seem that the court would benefit more from a clear statement as to the nature of the patient's illness and the manner in which it influences his behavior than from a conclusory statement which may have limited scientific validity. In most courts, however, the psychiatrist will find himself under considerable pressure to make definitive statements, particularly when litigation involves the competency of any involved parties.

What Is the General Legal Meaning of the Term "Incompetency"?

The issues of an individual's incompetency to stand trial and in-competency to elect or refuse treatment have been discussed in previous sections. In these forms of incompetency as well as in the forms to be considered here, the basic deficit of the incompetent person is his di-minished capacity to make or to communicate rational, self-serving deci-sions. Usually a person is found incompetent in order to protect him from the consequences of his own poor judgment. Sometimes, how-ever, there are socially expedient reasons for finding him incompetent. An individual, for example, may be found incompetent to make con-tracts or wills in order to protect his family or heirs. Or he may be found incompetent to be a witness in order to protect the parties in litigation.

In past decades there was some tendency automatically to consider patients who were severely mentally ill as incompetent.[1] As noted pre-viously, however, this is no longer true. Neither presence of mental illness nor the fact that a patient has been committed is sufficient reason these days to warrant an assumption of incompetency.[2] The current trend is in a direction of assessing an individual's competency to per-form specific functions. The patient's mental illness is relevant only insofar as it influences specific capacities. An individual might, for example, have a type of illness which influences his capacity to manage his business affairs, but does not influence his capacity to make a compe-tent decision as to whether to be given treatment. Or his mental illness might make him incompetent to perform certain contractual functions but not interfere with his capacity to make a will or serve as a witness. This functional approach to competency makes good sense. In past years committed patients or those adjudicated to be incompetent and in need of a guardian were deprived of many rights, including the right to vote, to sue, to marry, to obtain certain types of licenses, and to make contracts. Increasingly state laws are being changed to allow for specific determinations of incompetency so that an individual incompetent in one area can still retain his rights in other areas. The law has always held that all individuals are assumed to be competent until proven otherwise. Now the trend is to assume that the patient is competent in all areas in which he has not been specifically adjudicated incompetent.

The psychiatrist's task in incompetency proceedings is to determine if the patient has a mental disorder and whether that disorder may cause

[1]H. Davidson, *Forensic Psychiatry* (New York: Ronald Press, 1952).
[2]E. Z. Ferster, "Hospitalization and Incompetency," in *Mental Impairment and Incompetency*, edited by R. Allen, E. Ferster, and H. Weihofen (Englewood Cliffs, N.J.: Prentice-Hall, 1968).

a defect in judgment which compromises his capacity to make effective decisions in the matter in question. Sometimes, as in the case of incompetency to stand trial, the psychiatrist's testimony must be shaped to be responsive to specifically formulated standards. In other litigation, however, such as that involving determination of someone's competency to refuse treatment, the standards have not as yet been clearly defined.

What Issues Are Involved in Determining an Individual's Competency to Manage Business Affairs?

There are a number of mental illnesses which may seriously impair an individual's capacity to conduct certain types of business. Patients suffering from organic brain syndromes may have memory and orientation deficits serious enough to preclude their satisfactorily undertaking major commercial transactions. Patients with schizophrenic or affective psychoses may have similar difficulties. Families and friends of chronically sick patients are most likely to raise the issue of their financial incompetency. When an individual lacks the ability to know the extent of his material holdings or to handle his affairs wisely or prudently, he may be adjudicated to be incompetent to conduct business affairs. A guardian is then appointed (usually a family member or an attorney) who then makes the patient's financial decisions. In some states the determination of incompetency to conduct business affairs must be made under a "blanket" incompetency ruling which deprives the patients of many other rights. In other states a determination of incompetency to manage business affairs will not interfere with the patient's freedom to make decisions about other aspects of his life.

The psychiatrist's job in this type of incompetency proceeding is simply to determine if the patient is ill and how that illness might influence the patient's judgment in managing business affairs. Usually the psychiatrist finds himself testifying that a patient should be adjudicated incompetent, but he may also find himself arguing the reverse. Severe mental illnesses are often treatable, and over a period of time the patient's competency may be restored. The psychiatrist may then be employed to help the patient be adjudicated competent and to regain decision-making rights. State legislatures are increasingly aware of the need periodically to review the status of patients adjudicated incompetent.

Declaring an individual incompetent to manage his business affairs may be to that individual's benefit, but it may also be of considerable benefit to his heirs or acquaintances. They are likely to profit by more prudent management of the incompetent individual's estate. Some critics of forensic psychiatry argue that curtailment of a patient's autonomous power to conduct business affairs may primarily benefit others and be harmful to the patient.[3] They view many adjudications of incompetency as paternalistic infringements on the patient's rights. Certainly, the psychiatrist and the court should be alert to the possibility that the patient's level of incapacity is not great and that he might be more harmed by the adjudication of incompetency than by being allowed to conduct business affairs which are of questionably poor judgment.

What Are the Legal and Psychiatric Issues Involved in Determining Whether a Contract Can Be Voided on the Basis of One Party's Incompetence?

A contract may be made by two individuals who assume one another's competence, but one party may later seek to avoid fulfilling the contract on the grounds that he was incompetent at the time he made it. The party who claims incompetency is likely to seek the services of the psychiatrist to help prove the existence of his incapacity. In this situation there has usually been no prior adjudication of incompetence. The courts are faced with the task of making a retrospective determination of the patient's mental condition at the time the contract was made. There are similarities between this problem and the problem of determining whether an individual was insane at the time he committed a crime. It is not possible to examine a patient at the time of committing a crime or making a contract. The psychiatrist and the court must speculate as to an individual's mental status at some past moment by making inferences from historical data and by gaining insight from assessments of the patient's current mental condition.

In deciding whether to void a contract on the basis of a patient's mental illness, the courts must consider other difficult issues. Our free-enterprise society has a powerful interest in preserving the validity of contracts. At the same time, society has a *parens patriae* interest to protect the welfare of the incompetent patient. The patient's family also has some interest in ascertaining that their wealth is not dissipated frivolously. The Anglo-American courts have struggled with finding a just means of dealing with these conflicting interests for centuries.[4]

As the law in this area has evolved, several factors have come to favor voiding of the contract. One essential factor, of course, is the

---

[3]R. Leifer, "Competence of the Psychiatrist to Assist in the Determination of Incompetency," *Syracuse Law Review* 14 (1963): 564.

[4]H. Weihofen, "Mental Incompetence to Contract or Convey," *Southern California Law Review* 39 (1966): 211.

presence of a mental illness which impairs the patient's judgment. The courts generally rule that the contracting person must be capable of understanding the nature and consequences of the transaction. Sometimes this is worded as "did he know what he was doing and the nature of the act done?"[5] If the patient does not know the nature and consequences of his transaction, he may be viewed as insane. In some jurisdictions, an insane delusion test is utilized. If the patient has a false belief in the reality of facts and if this delusion may have motivated him to make a contract, the patient is likely to be considered incompetent.

Recently the courts have been concerned with the problems of patients with manic-depressive disorders who may understand the nature and consequences of their transactions but who in their driven manic state are likely to make irrational contracts. Under the traditional rules involving incompetency to contract such individuals are likely to be found competent. Courts have in recent years been trying to develop a test that would excuse the manic from contractual obligations. One ruling that has been proposed is that the contract will be considered to have been made by an incompetent person if the patient cannot behave reasonably with regard to the transaction and the other party to the contract has reason to know of his condition.[6] (Some legal scholars have noted that there is a shift in this direction from a specific cognitive test to a broader motivational test which in a rough way parallels the historic shift from *M'Naghton* to *Durham* in cases involving the plea of not guilty by reason of insanity.)

In addition to the patient's mental status at the time of the contract, there are other factors the court will consider in making a decision as to whether a contract is voidable. Where the other party had reason to suspect that the mentally disturbed individual was incompetent at the time the contract was made, the court is more likely to void. The contract is also more likely to be voidable if it is not deemed to be fair and reasonable. On the other hand the court is usually reluctant to void a contract unless the status quo with regard to money or property can be restored. An individual who was probably incompetent at the time of the transaction, but who cannot return the money or property obtained through the contract, may not be able to have the contract rescinded. As a general rule the courts are also unlikely to void a contract which involves purchases of necessities of everyday life such as food and clothing. Legal disputes involving efforts to rescind contracts on the basis of incompetency are probably diminishing. Our society is increasingly willing to allow people to return purchases if unsatisfied with their

---

[5]"Note, Mental Illness and the Law of Contracts," *Michigan Law Review* 57 (1959): 1020.
[6]Ortolere v. Teacher's Retirement Board, 250 N.Y.2d 196, 250 N.E.2d 640 (1969).

quality, and manufacturers are increasingly being required to assume responsibility for the quality of their products. These social and legal changes diminish the necessity to invoke mental disorder as a means of negating a contract.

On rare occasions the psychiatrist may be asked to testify on issues involving the patient's ability to fulfill rather than to make a contract. A severe mental illness, just like a severe physical illness, may limit or negate an individual's capacity to meet an obligation. An actor, for example, may become seriously disturbed after already contracting to appear in a film or a play. In testifying in this type of case the psychiatrist is asked to describe the nature and severity of the patient's illness and how it diminishes his capacity to perform specific tasks.

What Legal and Psychiatric Issues Are Involved in Determining an Individual's Competency to Make a Will?

The technical term for competency to make a will is "testamentary capacity." To have that capacity, a person making a will must: first, know that he is making a will; second, know the nature and extent of his property; and third, know the natural objects of his bounty. A defect in any of these three areas arising from a disease of the mind can negate the will. Obviously, some mental illnesses, and particularly organic brain syndromes, can produce a degree of confusion which diminishes an individual's capacity to meet any of the above criteria. A severely disturbed person might not even know he is making a will and might easily become confused as to the extent of his property and his natural heirs. People with mental illnesses which might not be accompanied by confusion can also have difficulty in meeting the criteria for testamentary capacity. Patients who have "insane delusions" or unrealistic beliefs as to the extent of their property, or as to who the natural objects of their bounty really are, may fail to meet testamentary capacity in terms of the second and third criteria.

In actual practice the mere existence of a psychosis or other mental illness does not in itself negate testamentary capacity. Patients can be extremely disturbed and still make a valid will if they meet the three traditional criteria. A will, at least in theory, does not have to be just or rational. The testator can be vindictive or frivolous, and can be plagued with a variety of other incapacities, but as long as he meets the above-noted criteria, his will is valid.[7]

---

[7]Davidson, *Forensic Psychiatry.*

The psychiatrist may be a witness for the party contesting the will or for the party hoping to sustain it. In either case the major problem for the psychiatrist in evaluating the competency of the person who made the will is that the individual is dead at the time the will is contested. The patient obviously cannot be examined, and it is extremely unlikely that the psychiatrist has ever had the opportunity to examine him. Here the psychiatrist is in the difficult position of having to determine the patient's mental status and how it relates to the three criteria for making a will on the basis of secondhand information. He must rely on someone else (usually the attorney of the client he is serving) to accumulate data as to the patient's behavior at the time the will was made. These data may include observations of others as to the patient's mental status, letters written by the patient, or medical reports. The psychiatrist must act more like a psychohistorian than a clinician. There is little room for certainty here, and the psychiatrist's conclusions may not have much greater validity than that of an educated layperson. A psychiatrist should anticipate rigorous cross-examination if he testifies on either side of this issue.

On rare occasions a psychiatrist may be asked to examine a patient who is making a will and attest to that person's competency. Here the psychiatrist's task is much easier. It is also possible that psychiatrists may have treated a patient whose will is being contested. If the treatment took place at the time that the will was made, the psychiatrist may again be able to contribute more relevant testimony as to the testator's competency.

There are certain social considerations involved in the determination of testamentary capacity of which the psychiatrist should be aware. Wills are usually contested by disinherited relatives who claim that their rejection in the will was caused by the mental illness of the testator. The courts tend to look carefully at the validity of a will which ignores the natural heirs, particularly if these heirs happen to be young children. In the latter situation society has a selfish interest in seeing that minor children receive some support from the deceased. Otherwise the state may have to assume financial responsibility for their welfare. The psychiatrist should also be aware that some critics of forensic psychiatry view use of expert testimony to negate wills as an aspect of social control.[8] They note that when the will meets society's generally accepted notions about what is right it is usually accepted, and that the psychiatrist is primarily used to provide medical rationalizations to negate wills which deviate from conventional social standards.

[8]T. Szasz, *Law, Liberty, and Psychiatry* (New York: Macmillan, 1963), pp. 72–78.

What Are Some of the Legal and Psychiatric Issues Involved in Determining the Competency and Credibility of Witnesses?

A good witness must be able to make observations, to recollect them, and to communicate his knowledge of them in court. He must possess these capacities with regard to the specific subject on which he is to testify. A wide variety of mental illnesses, and particularly organic brain syndromes, can impair these capacities. The actual determination of the individual's capacity to observe, recollect, and communicate is left to the judge, who may disqualify a witness on a motion of an attorney or by virtue of his own observation or knowledge. This is done away from the jury before the witness even takes the stand. Sometimes the judge may wish to call on the psychiatrist for help in making his decision. The psychiatrist then testifies as to how mental illness may impair the witness's capacity to observe, recollect, and communicate trustworthy evidence regarding the specific issue about which the subject is supposed to testify.

Once the witness is allowed to testify, the credibility of his testimony may be questioned. There is some belief in legal circles that the psychiatrist can, through a mental status examination, make useful observations about the witness's credibility. The judge has the option of ordering a psychiatric examination for certain witnesses, particularly those who may be making accusations. The credibility of accusers, particularly in sexual assault cases, is often in doubt, and on occasion judges' decisions have been reversed when they have failed to order psychiatric examination of the witness whose accusations were doubted.[9]

Some mental illnesses may influence the credibility of a witness's testimony. Psychotic individuals often distort their observations or may have difficulty in recollecting and communicating accurately. Patients with certain personality disorders may exaggerate, distort, or deliberately lie. There is no evidence, however, that psychiatrists have special skills in detecting when a given individual is providing mistaken information or is lying. The nature of our day-to-day work does not require such skills. When we are not sure about a patient's reliability, we try to obtain objective history from relatives, friends, or employers. In dealing with patients in psychotherapy, we anticipate that patients will distort reality but do not become too concerned about this because we assume that eventually the distortions will be clarified and that, through their examination, the patient's maladaptive defenses will be revealed. Psychiatrists may practice for weeks or months at a time without even

---

[9]R. Slovenko, "Witnesses, Psychiatry, and the Credibility of Testimony," *University of Florida Law Review 19*, no. 1 (1966).

questioning whether any of their pateints are telling the truth. For these reasons I believe that psychiatrists have developed few skills in detecting mendacity. Beyond providing generalizations as to how various kinds of mental impairments could contribute to the credibility of hypothetical witnesses, we have very little to contribute in this area.

The psychiatrist plays an especially dangerous game when he attempts to make observations about the credibility of witnesses he may not even have examined but has simply observed in the courtroom.[10] In the well-publicized trial of Alger Hiss, a prominent psychiatrist observed Hiss's accuser, Chambers, in the courtroom. On the basis of his observations and a certain amount of history of Chambers's behavior, the psychiatrist concluded that Chambers had a psychopathic personality disturbance and that his testimony was not credible. In this instance, the psychiatrist's testimony was in large part discredited by vigorous cross-examination and Hiss was convicted. Whether or not the psychiatrist in this case was right, he was not basing his testimony on scientific data or skills.

To What Extent Is Mental Illness a Factor in Determining an Individual's Liability for a Tort?

Like any other individuals, those who are mentally ill commit intentional or negligent torts. Although a physical disability may diminish the liability of a person who commits a tort, mental illness is rarely an excusing condition. The courts do not usually excuse the mentally ill tortfeasor because they are concerned that innocent victims need some remedy for changes even if the tortfeasor is ill. They are also concerned with the vagueness of the concept of mental illness and worry over the possibility that illness can be malingered. Finally, it is sometimes argued that holding the mentally ill responsible for torts may make their guardians more careful and alert. One of the few concessions provided in this area is that punitive damages are usually not allowed in a successful suit against a patient who is viewed as insane.

There have been a few instances in which the courts have negated liability for negligent torts. In cases where the court has judged that the patient could not foresee an "attack" of mental illness which played a role in his committing a negligent tort (such as an auto accident), the illness is treated somewhat like a physical illness and a subject may not be liable. Here, an "attack" of mental illness is viewed as somewhat

[10]"Note, Evidence—Courtroom Psychiatric Diagnosis—Valid or Invalid?" *Nebraska Law Review* 30 (1951): 513.

analogous to an attack of epilepsy. If the individual knew he was subject to epileptic attacks and drove anyway, he might be liable. If he did not know that he was susceptible to epileptic attacks (or "attacks" of insanity), he might not be liable. Psychiatric testimony could be used in this situation to delineate the manner in which mental illness played a role in the accident and to provide information as to the possibility that the "attack" was sudden and unanticipated.

The issue of the psychiatric status of the plaintiff in a tort suit may be of greater importance. One defense to a suit involving negligence is contributory negligence. If the plaintiff has conducted himself in a manner which falls below the standards to which he is required to conform for his protection, and if this conduct contributes as a legal cause to the harm he suffers, the defendant is not liable.[11] This is usually an "all-or-nothing defense" to a suit, and if contributory negligence can be proven, the plaintiff loses. The courts allow testimony regarding the insanity of the plaintiff to be introduced in arguing against the defendant's claim of contributory negligence. A patient with an organic brain disease may, for example, be careless with matches, may burn himself, and may sue the hospital. The defendants in this case may argue that the patient was contributorily negligent in violating instructions about not smoking. But the courts would probably hold in such a case that the patient was too confused or disoriented to follow instructions and could not be held accountable for contributory negligence. The tendency for the courts to allow insanity to negate contributory negligence partially accounts for the relatively infrequent use of this defense in malpractice suits involving psychiatric patients. There are no cases on record of a psychiatrist's successfully defending himself in a malpractice suit by claiming contributory negligence on the part of the patient.

How May the Psychiatrist Become Involved in Legal Issues Related to Marriage and Divorce?

Mental illness, or in legal terms "insanity," may be grounds for annulment of a marriage. It may be a defense to accusations of fault which lead to divorce, or it may be grounds for divorce.

Some people may be incompetent to enter into a marriage contract. If they lack the mental capacity to intend to marry or to comprehend the nature and consequences of the marriage ceremony, the marriage can be annulled.[12] Grossly intoxicated patients or those who suffer from con-

---

[11]W. Prosser, *The Law of Torts,* 4th ed. (St. Paul, Minn.: West, 1971).
[12]F. T. Lindman and D. M. McIntyre, *The Mentally Disabled and the Law* (Chicago: University of Chicago Press, 1961).

siderable confusion based on some other type of mental disorder might be incompetent to marry. Psychiatric testimony is on occasion invoked to substantiate this type of incompetency.

In many divorce cases the action is based on the fault of one of the parties. A spouse may be accused of cruelty, desertion, or adultery. The accused party may wish to disclaim fault and argue that he was not responsible for his behavior on the grounds that he was mentally ill. A patient, for example, involved in adulterous behavior might claim that he cannot be faulted for that act because he was mentally ill when the adultery took place. The psychiatrist's task here is similar to that involved in testifying in cases involving determinations of guilt or nonguilt for crimes by reason of insanity. Tests similar to the *M'Naghten* rule are applied. The psychiatrist is asked to reflect on the patient's mental status at some earlier time, and in effect assists the court in determining whether an individual should be held responsible for behavior which leads to divorce. [13]

In a number of states insanity can also be grounds for divorce. States which have statutes that allow divorce on the grounds of insanity usually require that the insanity be "incurable." Sometimes the law requires that the insane spouse must have spent a certain number of years in a mental hospital. Psychiatric testimony is sometimes called for here to ascertain the fact of the spouse's illness and to provide information as to its alleged incurability. Psychiatrists, of course, are uncomfortable in viewing mentally ill patients as "incurable" and are usually loathe to testify in these terms. One authority has argued that the standard of incurability should be changed to that of an "intractable, unremitting mental illness." [14]

What Is Required of a Psychiatrist Who Testifies in a Malpractice Suit?

Psychiatrists, like other doctors, are becoming somewhat less reluctant to testify as expert witnesses for a plaintiff in malpractice suits against a doctor, and certainly many psychiatrists are quite willing to testify as experts for their colleagues who are defendants. The psychiatrist who testifies for either side should be thoroughly familiar with the standards for diagnosis and treatment for the particular type of case involved. Sometimes the psychiatrist may only be asked to define duly careful standards of diagnosis and treatment. Here he functions primarily as an educator. More often, he will also be asked to determine the

---

[13]R. L. Sadoff, *Forensic Psychiatry: A Practical Guide for Lawyers and Psychiatrists* (Springfield, Ill: Charles C Thomas, 1975).
[14]*Ibid.*

extent to which the patient has been damaged and how such damage may have been caused by negligent treatment. The psychiatrist testifying for the plaintiff will usually be asked to provide data which support the thesis that duly careful standards were violated, that this did produce damage, and that the negligence was a necessary cause or cause in fact of the damages. The doctor testifying for the defendant may be called upon to argue that negligence did not occur, or that damage did not occur, or that if damage did occur it was not the result of negligent practice.

What Is the Role of the Psychiatrist in Suits Involving Civil Rights Actions?

Psychiatrists and psychologists have involved themselves in providing expert testimony in civil rights cases going back to the 1950s when the adverse psychological consequences of segregated school systems were described in desegregation suits.[15] Throughout the 1960s, psychiatrists and psychologists testified in right-to-treatment suits and helped to define the appropriate standards of care for mental hospitals.[16] This function has continued into the 1970s. A few psychiatrists have also made themselves available to patients resisting involuntary commitment and have viewed themselves as adversaries protecting their patients from unnecessary confinement. More recently, several psychiatrists have involved themselves as experts who have assisted the courts in cases where the constitutionality of commitment standards was in question.[17]

A psychiatrist can also assist prisoners in arguing that certain punitive practices are unconstitutional insofar as they are inherently dangerous to the prisoner's right to privacy or freedom to think, or are so psychologically painful as to be deemed cruel and unusual punishment. I have been involved in assisting plaintiffs in several suits against prison systems where the use of solitary confinement as punishment seemed to be inordinate and excessive. In these suits I simply provided information as to the possible psychological effects of prolonged sensory deprivation in an isolation cell. Partly on the basis of my testimony, the courts set limits on the conditions and length of solitary confinement.

It should be obvious that the psychiatrist who involves himself in a civil rights action usually takes some strong advocacy position on a

[15]Brown v. Board of Education, 347 U.S. 483, 74 S. Ct. 686, 98 L. Ed. 873 (1954).
[16]J. B. Robitscher, "Right to Psychiatric Treatment," *Villanova Law Review 18* (1972).
[17]"U.S. Court Upholds Danger Exam Standard," *Psychiatric News 13*, no. 13 (July 1978): 1.

political or moral issue. Because a psychiatrist is likely to be so heavily invested in the cause of the plaintiff, he should be exceptionally scrupulous and careful in providing relevant testimony. It is especially important that he separate fact from opinion and not make statements which pretend an expertise that does not exist.

16

Teaching Psychiatric Residents about Legal Issues

With all the new demands made by recent legal changes and with all the new interest in legal aspects of psychiatry, teaching about law in the practice of psychiatry remains surprisingly antiquated. Very few psychiatric residency training programs have expanded or changed their basic educational format in this area in the past decade. The majority of programs still continue to give a brief course on forensic psychiatry in the last year of training. Usually the content focuses on expert witness roles. The resident learns about issues involving malpractice and the treatment of severely disturbed patients largely through on-the-job training. Even departments of psychiatry with skilled forensic psychiatrists on their faculties do not provide residents with a great deal of teaching about legal issues. The forensic psychiatrist may be more involved in teaching courses on mental health law or other issues in the law school than in teaching about similar issues to residents. The law school course is usually too complicated or time-consuming to attract the interest of the psychiatric resident.

Educators who are interested in legal aspects of psychiatry have noted that residents tend to vacillate between being uninterested in the subject and being unduly alarmed by it. Many residents are bored with legal issues until they encounter a patient they want to treat but cannot, or until they are confronted with a situation which may involve a lawsuit. Most residents will see the theoretical issues involved in expert witness roles as somewhat esoteric and uninteresting until they become familiar with a patient who is involved in such litigation.

As a rule, the resident will have to encounter legal issues early in his training. In most programs the first-year resident deals with severely disturbed inpatients. He will soon find himself dealing with the issues of civil commitment, the patient's right to refuse treatment, and the need to initiate incompetency proceedings for patients who refuse treatment. The beginning resident, who is usually quickly introduced to the biological aspects of psychiatric treatment and litigious types of patients, may also encounter situations where he is threatened with a malpractice suit or is aware of the possibility of such a suit. This is especially true of the resident who works in the emergency room of a general hospital. For these reasons it would be helpful to bring some formal teaching with regard to the issues of malpractice and treatment of severely disturbed patients into the first year of psychiatric training. Currently such teaching is left to attending physicians and is not of uniform quality. Some attending physicians are interested in legal issues and enjoy teaching about them. Others view the legal regulation of psychiatry as they would a plague and try to indoctrinate the resident with as negative and defensive an attitude toward the legal system as is possible.

Beginning residents should receive at least three or four formal sessions on the basic issues involved in psychiatric malpractice, particularly as these relate to the creation of a duty in the emergency room and to the issue of the elements involved in obtaining consent to treatment. It is my belief that these issues can be presented in a way which will diminish the resident's fear of malpractice suits and will increase his respect for malpractice law as an instrument for improving standards of medical practice. The first-year resident should also learn more than just the mechanics of civil commitment and incompetency proceedings. A resident is more likely to participate in these proceedings in a manner which provides optimum benefits to his patient if he understands a little bit of the legal reasoning beyond the current attention to patients' rights and has a clear understanding of the limitations of his own role in this area. Too often beginning residents get seduced into taking an adversarial position with regard to the issue of civil commitment and begin to talk of "winning" or "losing" a commitment hearing. Such a view, which is both grandiose and legally incorrect, is eventually destructive to the resident's morale and can impair his clinical functioning. The beginning resident who has the opportunity to reflect on the philosophical issues involved in the civil commitment and incompetency proceedings will also make a better clinician. This type of instruction can be provided in a series of three or four sessions. Ideally, an attorney should participate in the seminars and present the legal arguments which lie behind the new restrictions.

I would also favor excusing first-year residents from participating in the commitment process. At this stage in their career they do not have enough experience in diagnosing and treating mental illness to exercise good judgment in initiating or sustaining a commitment petition. They often fear the prospect of testifying in court and usually make poor witnesses. Lacking an understanding of how commitment may help a patient, they can experience their participation in the process of depriving a person of freedom as psychologically devastating.

The teaching of expert witness roles can be left to later years of residency training. The psychiatric and legal issues involved in these roles are fascinating, but they are more likely to be appreciated by a resident who has already formed a reasonable identity of himself as a psychiatrist, feels some confidence in his clinical skills, and has the psychological equanimity leisurely to pursue exciting, intellectual issues. Residents are, of course, most likely to be interested in expert witness roles if the philosophical and legal issues can be directly related to clinical cases. It is possible to offer residents limited and closely supervised experiences as experts in certain types of criminal and civil proceedings. In some programs residents may evaluate patients for competency to stand trial. In most programs they testify in civil commitment hearings. It is difficult, however, to provide residents with the opportunity to testify in some of the more esoteric and complicated expert witness roles.

One way to help residents learn about all varieties of expert witness roles is to provide them with the opportunity to observe senior psychiatrists evaluate patients involved in criminal and civil litigation and then to observe that colleague's testimony in court. It is, of course, difficult to structure this kind of observational experience into a teaching curriculum, since the scheduling of cases cannot be at the convenience of residents. Nevertheless, programs should make efforts to provide advanced residents with sufficient time to observe closely those of their faculty who serve as expert witnesses. Those faculty members who become involved in expert witness roles usually do not combine these efforts with a teaching mandate. This is unfortunate. The experience of evaluating a patient and then testifying about that issue in court can be far more exciting and interesting to the expert when it is observed by students and later discussed with them.

While training in legal aspects of psychiatry need not be exhaustive or time-consuming, a few hours of didactic instruction and the opportunity to deal with or observe a number of cases involving legal issues seems essential to the training of a good psychiatrist. As long as psychiatric practice continues to be increasingly regulated by law, psychiatric educators have a responsibility to expand their trainees' knowledge of legal issues. As long as the legal profession continues to call upon psychiatrists to assume expert witness roles, psychiatric educators have a responsibility to ascertain that every graduate develop at least some capacity to function in these roles. Many psychiatrists will, of course, reject the role of expert witness whenever they can. They are certainly entitled to do this for personal or philosophical reasons. But it is especially unfortunate when they shun the role of expert simply because they have not been trained to assume it.

Index